PRAISE FOR THE BOOK SURVIVE AND THRIVE!
HOW CANCER SAVES LIVES

"The honest and inspirational stories of survival and the practical advice you and those you have interviewed give, will hopefully provide a roadmap for others to negotiate the difficult path you have followed."
— A/PROFESSOR ROBERT LINDEMAN, HAEMATOLOGIST, A/PROFESSOR, SCHOOL OF MEDICINE, UNIVERSITY OF NSW

"Jo Spicer's collection of inspirational stories of people who have had cancer should be compulsory reading for all health professionals who have any involvement in the care of people with cancer. Carefully balancing the harsh realities and the humour of cancer sufferers, Jo Spicer provides a window into the world of people who are facing a major threat to their lives. This book will contribute to better outcomes and a more holistic approach to cancer treatment. In addition to the many amazing stories, the book contains wonderful practical advice for cancer patients, families, and support persons. I salute the heroes of Survive and Thrive and thank Jo Spicer for her skill and dedication in bringing these stories to us."
— DR MARK BASSETT, EXECUTIVE DIRECTOR, MEDICAL SERVICES & CLINICAL GOVERNANCE, ILLAWARRA SHOALHAVEN LOCAL HEALTH DISTRICT, NSW HEALTH

"Jo has captured the essence and character of the people in this book beautifully. So much so that I feel like I sat round the kitchen table with them, fully involved in the discussions about their personal struggles with cancer. I am humbled by their generosity. Most experienced intense suffering, fear and seemingly insurmountable odds. Regardless or perhaps because of this, all exemplify how, in our darkest times, the human spirit can mobilise strength, determination, courage, hope and wisdom. While the individuals may not see this themselves, I believe they are incredible human beings who remind me of the dignity and preciousness of life."
— DR SUE LEICESTER, CLINICAL PSYCHOLOGIST

"In spite of a busy schedule, I genuinely had a lot of trouble putting Jo's book down. Too often as clinicians, we become largely-focused on the disease, as opposed to the person behind the condition. Their hopes, dreams, anxieties—this book provided a level of insight that I rarely have the chance to hear. Thank you, Jo for bringing together this remarkable collection of, not only survival, but in many ways success stories. I'm a better doctor for having read it."

— **DR MEGHAN DARES, ORTHOPAEDIC SURGEON**

"A truly remarkable collection of people's experiences and reactions facing the life-threatening condition that is cancer. Filled with wisdom and resources from those who know first-hand what it's like to face and survive a diagnosis."

— **EMELIE CARINÉ GUSTAVSSON, CANCERAID**

"I loved the book and I was impressed by the resilience of humans. I'm amazed at how people, who may not have considered themselves to be brave, are often very, very brave. I see people who are unable to cope with a stubbed toe, cope with life-ending illnesses and really find the strength in themselves that they didn't know was there. It seems a shame that people have to face the end of their life to realise what great depth of character they have. It was nice to read about the kindness that other members of the community were able to show to people who were in trouble. I hope it encourages other people not to be frightened to put out a helping hand to people who are unwell. Some members of the community feel uncomfortable when they see somebody without hair, or without a limb. They tend to withdraw but this is the time when people in trouble need all the help and support and kindness that they can get.

— **DR JENNY SMILEY, GP AND NATIONAL TELSTRA BUSINESS ZAFFYRE (SMALL BUSINESS) AWARD WINNER, 2006**

"This is such an honest insight into the effects of cancer from the very first signs through diagnoses and everything that comes after. Jo has captured the true spirit of the journey people go through on their fight to survive. How they come through it much wiser and stronger with a whole new outlook on life. I was captivated from the beginning of the book and hope that all cancer patients will get to read it. Nothing has been left out. It is a practical, no holds barred inspiring reference book on how to survive and thrive from a cancer diagnosis. Knowledge is power and the information in this book will empower whoever reads it."

— **MARALYN YOUNG, FOUNDER/PRESIDENT, BREAST AWARE**

"Within these pages, Jo and the people that have generously and bravely shared their stories give us a remarkable gift of knowledge, inspiration and hope. These are refreshing and empowering perspectives on how to approach a journey through cancer or indeed any other illness and to travel back to health and happiness. In sharing their experiences and insights, these heroes teach us how to live a better life. It is humbling and awe-inspiring and a great blessing."

— **DR APRIL TRAYNOR, FAMILY WELLNESS CHIROPRACTOR**

"What an inspirational and informative piece of literature! Unfortunately, people from all walks of life know someone who is suffering or has suffered through cancer. This is such a touching, yet practical approach to provide insight and hope for those who are facing this trauma. Well done, Jo."

—**DAVID CROWE, CEO, WOLLONGONG PRIVATE HOSPITAL**

"Couldn't put it down! The stories of how these amazing people have overcome the 'evil genius' are so inspiring. Having worked with clients who have been affected by cancer, the practical tips for patients and loved ones are priceless. Jo has a special gift of being able to connect with people on a very personal level, providing readers with greater insight into how to not only survive, but to thrive!"

— **DIANNE CHALK, CERTIFIED FINANCIAL PLANNER, AGED CARE SPECIALIST**

"A warm and very human collection of stories from everyday heroes whose transformation, as a result of their cancer journey, proves that what we often fear as crisis, can indeed be a gift. You will be richer for this experience."

— **KYM KREY, BUSINESS MENTOR, LEADERSHIP SPECIALIST**

SURVIVE AND THRIVE! HOW CANCER SAVES LIVES

INSPIRING STORIES FROM COURAGEOUS
CANCER THRIVERS

JO SPICER

CROWN KENT

Published by Crown Kent

In conjunction with GOKO Management and Publishing

PO Box 7109, McMahon's Point 2060, Sydney, Australia

Library in Congress Cataloguing-in-Publication Data

Spicer, Jo

Survive and Thrive! How Cancer Saves Lives: True stories of cancer survivors providing inspiring and practical information to help patients and caregivers to thrive.

LCCN: 2018911687

ISBN: 978-0-6484361-0-2

Disclaimer:

The information and opinions expressed in this book are based only on the personal experience of the author and the information provided to the author by the people interviewed for this book. The author is not a medical practitioner of any kind and the book is not intended as a medical guide or manual. It is not designed to provide diagnosis or treatment or any type of professional medical advice. If you or any other individual chooses to take any recommendations from this book, please do not do so before consulting your health care professionals.

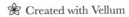 Created with Vellum

To the courageous cancer thrivers
who have shared from their hearts
to help others to Survive and Thrive!

CONTENTS

FOREWORD

CANCER IS A JOURNEY AND THERE ARE MANY PATHS TO BE TAKEN. Each cancer patient, their carers and family members, take different paths. The important message to take from this book is that there are no right or wrong paths. You may be given information on the hospital and treatment regimens, but each person's journey and experience is individual, personal, and profoundly life-changing.

Jo Spicer brings the stories of some of those who have taken this journey. Her own cancer journey makes her highly qualified to relate their stories. She tells them with clarity, energy, humour and compassion. She does not hide the hard facts or losses of those who have taken up the challenge and not only survived but thrived.

They may not have willingly embraced all the changes that a cancer diagnosis brings to all levels of a person's life, but they have created their own meaning and purpose. Priorities are changed, friends are lost, and new ones found. Physical and emotional scars form part of the whole. No one escapes unchanged.

It is significant that the final part of the book includes a section titled "For The Primary Support Person: How To Cope As a Caregiver." So often the carer is overlooked. Their journey can be as difficult, and sometimes more difficult than that of the patient with feelings of confusion, helplessness and fear. Drawing on her own personal experience and those of the survivors featured in this book, Jo's practical "Do's and Don'ts" do indeed give some guidance for the carer to survive and thrive as they enter this unknown territory.

These stories do not offer a recipe for success. Rather, they pay homage to the challenges and rewards, the pain and joys as lives are impacted by a diagnosis of cancer. There may be some readers who cannot relate to these stories and whose own journey has ended differently. But what can't be ignored is that for those who take the journey, life and death will be viewed differently. There will be those on the fringes who will never understand the travails of the journey, often the true impact is hidden. The important message is that each reader honours their own journey.

Professor Liz Lobb
PhD, M App Sci, B. Adult Ed.
Psycho-oncology and Palliative Care Researcher
Bereavement Counsellor, Sydney

INTRODUCTION

CANCER IS A WORD THAT INVOKES A MUCH GREATER MEANING than its dictionary definition. Type "what is cancer?" into your search engine and the answer you will find will be some variant of "a disease of the cells," or "a disease in which abnormal cells divide uncontrollably." These definitions are certainly correct, but this simple word is imbued with dramatic connotation.

The mere mention of cancer conjures up thoughts of terminal illness, death and horrific treatment. Whether your experience of cancer is personal, or as a friend or caregiver of someone who has had cancer, or even if you are the rare individual who has not personally come into contact with a cancer patient, you will undoubtedly have heard about someone who has fought the disease.

Worse still are the emotions and traumatic memories we connect to cancer. If someone drops the word into a conversation, it is impossible not to think of someone who has suffered at the hand of this "evil genius." This is my favourite nickname for cancer, borrowed from my doctor friend who described to me how effective and clever cancer is at compromising our bodies—it made me think of a villain from a superhero movie! Cancer is now so much a part of our vernacular that we use it to describe any malignant or destructive phenomenon.

Before I experienced cancer myself, I shared these thoughts. My grandmother died of cancer when I was 18 and she was the only person I knew who had the disease. In my mind, cancer equalled death. A lot has changed since then, and the last 30 years have brought about significant breakthroughs and advancements in technology and research. That old equation is no longer true, with more and more people receiving treatment and surviving.

According to the World Health Organisation (WHO) figures released in February 2018, there were 14 million new cases of cancer in 2012. WHO estimates that this number is expected to rise by about 70% over the next two decades. WHO also reported that in the same year, 2012, cancer accounted for 8 million deaths. These figures suggest that around 45% of cancer patients are surviving.

This information and my own cancer experience led me to ask questions about why some people survive and why others do not. Is it purely the result of researchers and scientists developing new ways to deal with the 'evil genius'? Does a person's mental attitude play a part in their ability to overcome the disease? How does the support of family and friends impact on the recovery process? Do newly diagnosed cancer patients find it reassuring or hindering to gain knowledge and information about their disease? Does a person's emotional state have any bearing on the success of the treatment of their physical body?

These questions sparked further curiosity to discover how a person's life is impacted and changed through the life-threatening trauma of cancer. Why do some people seek to return as quickly as possible to the normalcy of their pre-cancer lives, whilst others tend to adopt profoundly altered ways of thinking and new directions in life as a result of their experience with cancer?

In order to explore these concepts, I am honoured to share the stories of 31 beautiful people who have travelled on their own cancer journeys. These stories are not just of survival—remaining alive after an event—but of people who have thrived—flourished, prospered and grown—as a result of their cancer experiences. They are people of all ages ranging from three to 76 years, and they have all triumphed over different types of cancer. Some of them have done it more than once.

I am forever grateful for their frankness and willingness to share the darkest and the brightest parts of their journey, with the sole purpose of helping others.

The majority of the people in this book are Australian, as am I, so I have used Australian spelling and language. I have also included a terminology index at the back of the book to explain medical references.

For cancer patients, I invite you to let the stories inspire and motivate you. Learn from their experiences, choices and actions. Gain first-hand knowledge to ensure you make the best possible decisions for your own treatment and care.

For supporters and caregivers, I ask you to read with the aim of embracing your role. I hope that you gain invaluable insight into what your loved one or friend is thinking and feeling. Understanding their trauma assists you in providing the support that will help them the most.

For those of you who have not dealt with cancer, I urge you to think about the challenges that life has put before you. It could be a different kind of illness, or a confronting work situation. You may be struggling financially, or with a relationship or family drama. The stories you read here aspire to help you find your way through the darkness and to overcome adversity. Discover clarity and hope to light your way. Be motivated by these everyday heroes and let their wisdom speak to your heart and lift you higher.

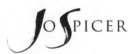

1

RENAE

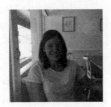

DIAGNOSIS: HODGKIN'S LYMPHOMA STAGE 4

Renae is a delightful 33-year old with everything to live for. Her engaging smile and warmth convey an inner strength and grace, qualities which she has developed through her incredible journey.

Following the path of many young Australians, Renae decided to begin her working life overseas. After graduating from University as a High School Teacher, she worked in casual positions in the UK and enjoyed living and working abroad for several years.

In her late twenties, Renae decided to return home and get serious about her future goals of finding a permanent teaching position and to buy her own home.

Everything seemed to be going to plan: Renae secured a one-year contract at the prestigious Illawarra Grammar School and she moved home to live with her Dad to help save up for a property deposit.

It was a wonderful experience. Renae was well-loved by her peers and students, her natural caring and mentoring approach so valued by those around her. The position proved to be the perfect springboard to achieve her ultimate goal as she successfully secured a permanent position at another school for the following year.

Renae had always been active and healthy, so when a few odd health issues popped up, she did not think they were anything to worry about. Renae thought that she was too young for any dreadful diseases.

It started with a niggling pain in her back that would not go away. Thinking she had pulled a muscle or strained something, Renae went to an osteopath and thought that the treatment had made her better.

Then with three weeks left until the end of current teaching contract, Renae started a pattern of coming home from work and sleeping for two to three hours in the afternoon, getting up to eat some dinner, and then going back to bed. She was totally exhausted all the time but attributed it to a really busy year working full-time.

"You self-diagnose and think, I'm tired, maybe it's glandular fever. I've got a pain in my back, maybe it's a pulled muscle."

Then a lump appeared out of nowhere on Renae's neck. She thought that she had swollen glands. Eventually it was her Dad who pressed her to see a doctor as there was obviously something wrong. So Renae went along to her GP for blood tests, not particularly concerned about the outcome.

Things were a little different when she went back for the results the following week. Renae's GP said that she needed to see a haematologist the next morning. Renae left her GP's office none the wiser as she had never heard of a haematologist and needed to Google the term. Even when she found out that a haematologist was a blood specialist, her mind did not go to a cancer diagnosis. In hindsight, she realises that her thinking was a little naïve.

Everything changed for her the next day. The haematologist took one look at the lump on her neck and told her that it was probably lymphoma. There was one other condition it could possibly be, but he thought it unlikely. Renae was immediately booked in for a biopsy to confirm his diagnosis.

This news gave Renae time to prepare her thinking. Even though her parents are divorced, her family is very close, and she was able to talk with them about the possibility of a cancer diagnosis.

After the surgery, her tissue was tested, and she underwent a PET scan. The haematologist confirmed that Renae had Stage 4, Hodgkin's Lymphoma. Hearing Stage 4 sent her into a panic.

"I remember being in complete shock. This was really serious! My first thought was, 'Am I going to die? Is this real? How can this be real?'"

Renae is thankful for the way her haematologist put her at ease. He reassured her that this was a type of cancer that could be treated, and that Stage 4 was an indication of spread, not severity. Her diagnosis was no better or worse than a Stage 1 or 2 diagnosis, it was simply to indicate that there were lesions in more than one site. For Renae, the cancer was in her neck, below the abdomen and in her spleen.

It was also a blessing that Renae's older sister, Olivia, attended this appointment with her. Olivia had been living in the Northern Territory at the time, but just happened to be home that week. Their parents were both unavailable that day, so it was fortunate Olivia was there. Renae recalls just sitting in the doctor's office freaking out, while Olivia asked all the questions.

The next steps were a complete whirlwind. Renae was sent off to the surgeon that same day. She was booked in for surgery to have the lump removed the following week and was also scheduled to commence chemotherapy within three weeks.

It all happened so quickly, and at a critical time of the school year. Renae remembers going back to work for the remaining three weeks of term, and instead of receiving a fond farewell and good wishes for her new position, it became a strange mix of emotions when she shared that the position was on hold because she was going to be having chemotherapy for a serious cancer.

"I remember them all being really worried and very concerned. Because I wasn't coming back the following year, so many of them touched base during my treatment to see how I was going. Such lovely people."

To complicate matters further, Renae had just started dating Rick around the time of her diagnosis. They had actually known one other all their lives, growing up two houses from each other. They lost touch when Renae moved overseas and only reconnected once she returned. The couple was in the early stages of their relationship, and Renae remembers the thoughts running through her head at the time:

"I hope he's not staying in this because I'm sick, because it would be really awful to break up with someone while they are having chemo. I hope he's just not hanging around because it would be bad timing for me."

As it turned out, Renae did not have to worry. Their relationship was genuine and even though it seemed like it progressed quickly, they were never concerned that they were moving too fast. It felt right, probably because of their long history together.

The strength of their relationship proved to be an important factor in the decision that Renae had to make regarding her treatment. Her haematologist provided two chemotherapy drug options and outlined the pros and cons for each.

The first option offered a 90% success rate in killing the cancer, first time. The downside of this drug, however, was that it would virtually guarantee that she would not be able to have children.

Option two had a 75% success rate but offered a slim 10% chance of being able to conceive. Aged just 29 and in a new relationship, Renae was forced to make a life-determining decision. She had always wanted to have children, but up until that point, she had lived as so many people in their twenties do: travelling, working and enjoying life, resting easy with the knowledge that there was plenty of time to have babies and settle down in the future.

"I was sitting there, thinking maybe I should have been thinking about these things sooner because now I am faced with the possibility of not being able to have a family. I was really gutted."

After serious conversations with her then boyfriend, Rick and her family, Renae opted for option two, offering the better chance of having children in the future. She began six months of chemotherapy in two weekly cycles. Each Friday fortnight she was infused with the chemotherapy drugs and a steroid medication which caused her to bounce off the walls with energy over the weekend.

The following Monday and Tuesday she would flatline, and then by Wednesday her energy would be at its lowest point leaving her feeling awfully unwell. From Thursday and over the following seven days, Renae would gradually build back her strength, ready for the cycle to begin all over again the next day. Fortunately, she did not feel nauseous, but her other main side effect was the complete loss of hair.

"Going to oncology every Friday fortnight was awful. But then I would think about all the other people in there having chemo as well. I would tell myself, it's not just you. It could actually be much worse."

Being well known in the community, Renae was blessed to be supported and wished well by friends and so many people wanting to do nice things. Renae's childhood friend, Alex Woods, was so shocked by Renae's diagnosis that she wanted to do something to support her friend. Through a Facebook campaign, Alex shaved her head and raised over $30,000 for the Cancer Council. This really helped to buoy Renae's spirits during treatment.

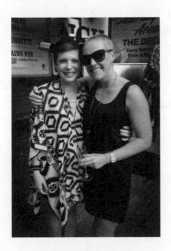

Renae & Alex

Throughout her treatment, Renae actually thought she was doing well, but on reflection, looking at photos of herself, she now realises that she was pale, washed out and very sick despite her constant reassurances to her family that she was going to be alright. Olivia kept buying her beautiful headscarves as her way of being useful and she recalls wondering why they all kept fussing over her. Looking at those photos helped her to understand how difficult it must have been for her family to see her in that state.

Renae's entire family was very supportive and Olivia actually moved back permanently. Living at home with her Dad meant Renae did not have to worry financially, and her new employer was happy to delay her start date by six months. Not having to worry about these things alleviated a lot of pressure.

"I seemed to spend a lot of time reassuring other people. In some ways it was a good coping mechanism, because when I said to other people, I'm going to be okay, it was like an affirmation, so in some ways it was good, in other ways it was exhausting."

Half way through chemotherapy, Renae was advised to see a fertility specialist. As a couple, she and Rick were forced to talk about the subject of family planning very early on in their relationship.

The chemotherapy treatment was completely successful, so immediately after, Renae began the In Vitro Fertilisation (IVF) process. She began having hormone injections and hoped to have her eggs frozen, however her Anti-Mullerian Hormone (AMH) reading was very low. For Renae, this was a major blow.

They went ahead and did one round of IVF regardless of the AMH reading and it was a failure. An ultrasound revealed that there were not enough eggs in there to retrieve. They were told that it was normal and sometimes it takes a few rounds. This all happened towards the end of the year near Christmas, so Renae decided to give it a break and leave the next round to the new year.

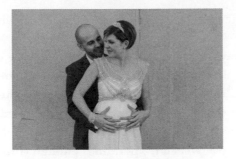

Rick and Renae on their wedding day

After such an emotionally draining period, Renae and Rick deserved a joyous Christmas, and as it happened, their gift was a miracle named Stella! In January, they discovered that there was no need for IVF, they had fallen pregnant naturally. They decided to get married, and four months later, Stella was born, a beautiful, healthy miracle.A few years later, Renae and Rick felt lucky to conceive their son Leo naturally. At his 20-week scan, the sonographer left the room to call in a doctor, and Renae recalls saying to Rick, "That's not good". Once they returned, she could sense from the way they were engaging that there was something wrong. It was there they were told that Leo had a heart defect.

For her entire pregnancy, Rick and Renae were terrified of what was going to happen when he was born. They had already overcome big hurdles as a couple, and these experiences had developed their resilience. They realised that they were made of "pretty tough stuff" and always maintained hope, telling themselves that it would be okay, because it had to be.

Their beautiful boy was delivered and underwent open heart surgery soon after. Leo and his family virtually lived in the hospital for his first three weeks. It is hard to imagine what those weeks would have been like. Renae remembers saying to Rick:

"That's what the cancer was for. To prepare us. In the grand scheme of things, it makes the six months of chemo feel really insignificant when compared to our newborn having major surgery."

The days after Leo's surgery were the most harrowing:

"We kept saying, 'He's going to be fine, we're going to get through it. It's going to be hard, but we'll be alright.' I really think this helped us when we were in the Children's hospital for those three weeks. It was so stressful, we were sleep deprived, spending every minute with him, feeling guilty that we weren't spending enough time with our daughter. But with all these challenges, at the same time we were thinking, 'We've got this.'"

Surgery was successful; Leo has a cute zipper scar on his chest and is as strong and brave as the lion for which he was named. Renae feels so blessed to have her beautiful family and is looking forward to teaching again. If they have another child, that would be a bonus. Right now, they are happy, hopeful and positive about their future.

"It's absolutely okay to freak out. It's alright to be scared, to be terrified because it's a real thing and your fears are justified. But at the same time, it's okay to be hopeful and positive, in fact it's absolutely necessary."

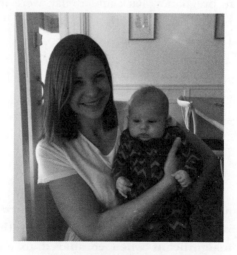

Renae and Leo

2

CARL

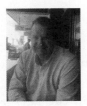

Representing your country as an Olympian is the pinnacle of achievement in any athlete's career. As spectators, we marvel at their incredible feats and think little of the years of physical and mental training that determined a medal winning performance.

When Carl, an Olympic swimmer, was diagnosed with testicular cancer, it was those years of becoming an elite athlete that shaped the positive attitude he needed to win back his life.

As we sipped coffee in Carl's local area, the Eastern Suburbs of Sydney, I noticed that every few minutes someone would wave as they walked by. Some would stop for a brief chat. Carl was welcoming and kind; I saw that it was not his background, but his genuine interest and care for people that has forged these friendships.

I asked Carl to tell me about his early life, and it was immediately evident why he rose to the top echelon of his sport—failure did not discourage him, it simply fuelled him to do better.

Carl grew up in the southern suburbs of Sydney. To keep him busy and out of mischief, his parents enrolled him into a local Saturday afternoon swimming club. Carl was 13 at the time, and the coach suggested he do some training to improve his performance. The hard work paid off because when Carl turned 14, he managed to make the national qualifying time.

This took him to the state championships where he made the national time by 0.1 of a second. This result allowed him to go to the nationals, where he came last.

"Getting last spurred me on. I thought I had better keep training a bit harder."

The following year Carl swam at the nationals in the 15/16 age group and came fifth. He returned the next year and won the race.

"A lot changed between the ages of 14 to 16. Everything changed: my attitude, my training, everything."

It was now 1984, and Carl went to the Olympic trials at age 16 and came last in the trials final. Again, this drove him to improve. Two years later, he qualified for the Commonwealth Games in Edinburgh, bringing home a bronze medal. Two years later, Carl qualified for the 1988 Seoul Olympics, reaching the finals in the 4 x 100m relay.

"I could have said at 14, this is probably the fastest I will ever go, and that could have been it. But if you open your mind and open your eyes and believe that something better can happen, it usually does."

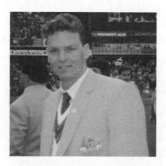

Carl in his official Games Blazer

This strong mental attitude played a major part in helping Carl through the greatest challenge of his life.

It started when Carl noticed his testicles were swollen and painful. He was 36 at the time and found that every afternoon he would come home from work and feel the need to lie on the couch icing them. This went on for around two weeks. Carl thought that one of his kids had accidentally hit him, but he could not remember an incident. Eventually, the swelling increased to the point where Carl's wife, Barbara, urged him to go to the doctor.

His GP referred him to a urologist, and Carl recalls thinking, "Another doctor...I don't have time for this." Carl and Barbara were running their own successful real estate agency with seven staff employed—all he could think about was getting back to work.

Two days later the urologist booked him in for a fine needle biopsy and Carl remembers watching the operation thinking, "This is quite possibly the worst thing that you could ever have happen." I imagine any man's eyes would water at the mere thought of having such a procedure done.

The urologist called Carl back the next day and quite factually told him that he had cancer. He added that it had probably been developing for a while, and that it was serious. The main concern was the extent of spread as the cancer had already travelled to the top of his spermatic cord. The doctor was unsure if it had entered his stomach.

Carl had surgery, and then started chemotherapy straight away. His regime was to be four cycles spaced at three-week intervals, however problems with infection resulted in the treatment process being drawn out with delays.

At the time of Carl's diagnosis, Barbara was pregnant with their third child, Laura.

"I don't know how Barbara made it through, but she did. She's very strong. Laura's strong too. She was born under stress and duress and that's probably part of it. She needed to be strong and determined to get on the ground."

Barbara was not only pregnant, but also trying to keep the business afloat, which proved to be extremely difficult. As with most small businesses, if there is no one bringing in clients, there is no income, and this makes it impossible to meet expenses.

"We didn't have any insurance, so at this point we had to dig in. The rental properties were not covering the wages and we were going backwards."

The family faced pressure from everywhere: Carl dealing with a life-threatening cancer; Barbara having to add the role of business manager to her already full load as wife, carer, mother and expectant mother; their two older children wondering what was happening to Dad; their business struggling to stay solvent; and the financial stress of meeting their commitments.

When you are diagnosed with cancer, the shockwaves ripple out to every area of your life. No one is ever fully prepared for it, but Carl realised that the years of discipline and training he went through as a teenager could help him to handle the crisis that he now faced.

"I always looked on the bright side. I probably credit swimming with that. Coming last in races and getting beaten by boys and girls in the same age group made me resilient!"

Carl recalls the times he sat in hospital and said to Barbara, "The guy next door to me is in a lot of trouble." She would agree, but think to herself, "It's not so good for you either."

There was never a moment that Carl entertained a negative thought about his own prognosis. He knew the success rate was high. Carl had three friends who had successfully beaten the same cancer, so he held the firm belief that he would "make it out" too.

"After three months of chemo, I'm bald and I go straight back to work because I didn't have any other option. I didn't have time to stop and get better. I treated it as though it didn't happen and just went on with my life."

After chemotherapy, Carl's doctor was satisfied that no further treatment was necessary. From this point on, all Carl needed to do was to show up for a CT scan every three months.

Everything was fine for the first three scans, but the fourth scan, which happened to be on the anniversary of his original diagnosis, showed a reoccurrence. The news was devastating.

Carl went to the Prince of Wales Hospital and he tells me that his oncologist looked absolutely miserable when he delivered Carl's diagnosis. He explained that because the cancer had returned and also spread to his stomach, Carl was in serious trouble and required aggressive treatment. He suggested that in hindsight, they should have administered higher doses or more rounds of chemotherapy the first time in view of Carl's tall swimmer's build.

His new regime was set for 10 rounds of chemotherapy at intervals of three weeks. The plan was to finish just before Christmas so that Carl could take a break from treatment over the holiday period, before starting on a radical new treatment in the new year.

Carl was one of the first patients to undergo the treatment protocol of high-dose chemotherapy followed by stem cell rescue. His oncologist, Professor Friedlander, Director of Medical Oncology at the Prince of Wales Cancer Centre, worked together with Associate Professor Lindeman, leading Haematologist at Prince of Wales Hospital, to administer the treatment protocol to save Carl's life.

In preparation for the treatment, after his ninth round of chemotherapy, Carl was connected to an apheresis machine which received his blood and separated it into its components of plasma, platelets, white blood cells and red blood cells. The plasma was saved for Carl's future treatment and the other components were returned to his body.

On completion of his tenth and final round of regular chemotherapy, Carl enjoyed four weeks off to recuperate and spend time with his family over Christmas.

During that time, he was relaxing and watching TV when a documentary screened featuring Professor Robert Tindle and his daughter Danielle. The program told the amazing story of Professor Tindle's breakthrough discovery back in the 1980s that led to the use of stem cells to save thousands of lives around the world. It also made possible the treatment that was used on his own daughter.

Carl could not believe it when Danielle described the exact treatment he would be undergoing in a matter of days. She talked about how the high-dose chemotherapy stripped the lining from her mouth and all the way through her stomach and to her gut causing nausea, vomiting and bleeding from every orifice. The toxicity was so high that her liver failed. Her oncologist said she was as close to death as you can get before the stem cell transplant gradually began working, with scans showing that her tumour was 100% gone.

This scenario was playing in Carl's mind as he was asked, prior to the procedure, to sign a waiver freeing the hospital of any liability.

"It seemed a lot worse than normal chemo. We were going next level. It sounded awful and I was really not looking forward to it."

Carl was set up in an isolation room to completely segregate him from any possibility of infection. No visitors were allowed—the only people to enter the room were his medical team, suited up in gowns, masks and gloves. Carl's family had to wave at him through the glass window.

The high-dose chemotherapy made him extremely sick. Carl was closely monitored over the next two weeks as he progressively deteriorated to his lowest point. When his white cell count was virtually nil, his harvested stem cells were then re-introduced, and he slowly started to improve. He remained in the isolation room for around five weeks before being allowed to go home.

Carl and Barbara realised that his recuperation would take some time.

"We had to make some drastic decisions. We'd gone back a fair way on the mortgage. We were really struggling, getting to a situation where we couldn't keep employees, so we had to let them go. We sold the rent roll to a friend, not for top dollar, but so both the tenants and the landlords were looked after. That gave us a little bit of money that allowed us to hang in there for the 18 months it took me to recover."

Cancer crashed the family's financial situation and the business they had worked so hard to build. Not only was Carl's life in danger, so too was their livelihood and all their plans for the future. Even now, 13 years later, they are still working hard to come back from it. Carl's illness had a dramatic impact on all the relationships in his life.

"It really affected the children, they see the physical changes like Dad has no hair and no eyebrows...they didn't know if I was going to be around. It affected everyone. My wife wasn't sure whether I was going to make it through. One hopes for the best, I was certainly positive, but she wasn't so sure it was going to be okay."

The treatment was a success. Today Carl is healthy and well. His journey has caused him to reprioritise his life. His three children, Jack, Lily and Laura are now the central focus of his life. Jack and Laura are great swimmers and Carl loves to watch them train and compete.

"My kids are pretty tough, they're strong and they quite like swimming. It teaches them teamwork and goal setting. I've met some really tough people in swimming, not outwardly tough, but inside."

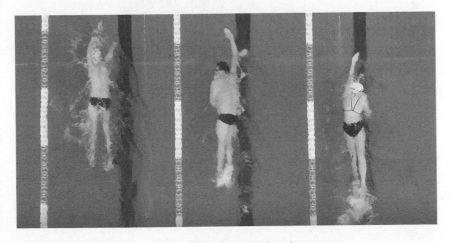

Jack, Carl and Laura in the pool

Carl has also changed his outlook on living a good work-life balance. Rather than working 24 hours a day and stressing over his own business, Carl is still in real estate, but now works for an agency.

"The family is really important to me and seeing them achieve and succeed and be positive and learn lessons is more important than huge financial success."

These days Carl counteracts life's stress and pressure by taking time to enjoy the sunshine. He takes 10 minutes to drive past the beach and breathe the refreshing salt air. He stops to chat with people and brightens the day of everyone around him. In his own words, **"I'm alive and that's a super-positive thing!"**

"When you find yourself in a situation like this, some people deal with it well and some people don't. The ones with the positive outlook are the ones who get through. My mental attitude was good—it's how you think that makes the difference."

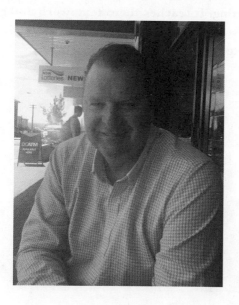

3

LUCIANA

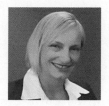

Diagnosis: Breast Cancer Her2 Positive

Luciana is a force of nature. From our very first conversation, I sensed her passion for life and the people around her. Lou, as she is known by most, is a rare and incredible woman who never lets anything hold her back from being her best self.

The daughter of immigrant Italian parents, Lou was raised with the values of many first-generation Australians. Her parents arrived in their new adopted country with nothing, working hard to create a better life for their children. Lou started a degree in languages but gravitated to law and today she is a successful and highly respected family law specialist.

In December 2007, Lou opened her own practice with colleague and now business partner, Tiana. Establishing the new firm took an incredible amount of focus and dedication. The two women, together with Lou's husband Rob, their accounts manager, worked tirelessly to get the practice off to a brilliant start.

Just three months later, Lou, aged 44, noticed a lump in her breast. Because her mother had experienced breast cancer seven years prior,

Lou was well aware of the possible implications and within two days she was at the Breast Cancer Clinic.

"I knew before I got there that it was cancer. I told my husband and he kept saying, 'No, no, no, you'll be fine.' And I said, 'I just get the feeling that it's cancer.' I was already mentally prepared for it."

The mammogram of Lou's breast did not show any abnormalities, but the doctor could feel the lump and proceeded with an ultrasound. He told her that if, on a scale of one to five, one being a cyst and five being cancer, he rated her at around a three.

"I thought, 'Well then, it's not a cyst, so therefore it can only be cancer.'"

To make a definitive diagnosis, Lou had a fine needle biopsy which showed that she had a malignant cancer. A core biopsy was taken immediately following this discovery and it confirmed that she had breast cancer. Lou left the clinic five hours later with a calm perspective on her diagnosis.

"My mother had breast cancer and it didn't kill her. I know other people who had breast cancer. Kylie Minogue had just been diagnosed around the same time, so I had a celebrity connection. I knew I'd got to it early. I was positive. I knew it wasn't the end of the world."

Her first phone call was to Rob who was away on a mountain-bike weekend with their son, Christian. He offered to come back, but Lou said no, she would wait until they returned.

"I told my sister Teresa. She cried, she screamed and was totally hysterical. I also phoned Tiana and she was the same. I had to calm them both down. Then I couldn't tell my kids. It was a hard weekend. I just didn't tell anybody or talk about it. On the Sunday night I told our daughter.

The drama and the hysteria! I was calm, I had to calm them all down."

Lou went on the internet to search for information on her diagnosis and treatment. Being armed with knowledge and experience gave her the confidence to expect a good outcome. But what impact would the treatment process have on her business? What if she had to have a lot of time off? How long would the treatment take? These were pressing questions that she needed answered.

On the Monday morning, Lou saw the surgeon who told her she would need a lumpectomy and radiation. The procedure was scheduled for the following week and Rob intended to drive her to the hospital.

It all became a bit more complicated when Rob did some mountain bike stunts on a ramp in his mate's backyard. He fell off his bike, broke his elbow and needed surgery. This was just three days before Lou's lumpectomy. Rob told his doctor that surgery would have to wait until after his wife's breast cancer surgery and this resulted in Lou driving herself to hospital with Rob and his bandaged arm as a passenger.

On the day of surgery, Lou's first attended the Prince of Wales Hospital to have the dye injection for her lymphoscintigram. Once this was done, Lou then drove herself and Rob to St Luke's Hospital for her surgery. She laughs as she tells me how they were greeted:

"We arrived, and they looked at Rob and said, 'Sir, how can we help you?' And I go, 'No, no, it's not him!' Even on my day, my time to shine, he stole my thunder!"

Prepped and ready to be wheeled to theatre, Lou recalls this as her worst moment. The doctor said, "Everything's looking good, but when we open you up, that can be a different thing. If it's worse than I think it is, I won't just lop off your breast and tell you after. You come out and we will tell you what has to be done."

Being told that the surgery was not necessarily going to solve the problem and that things might be worse than she had been led to believe was something that Lou did not want to hear—it was the one time that she was really upset.

Post-surgery, the news was not good. Lou's doctor scheduled her for a second surgery, to go back in and cut wider margins. This took place two weeks later.

The removed tissue was tested, and Lou was informed that she was HER2 positive. This type of breast cancer grows quickly and aggressively; but on the flip side, these cancer cells are also highly reactive to the right drugs.

Lou's treatment regime began with chemotherapy just six weeks after surgery. The timing was not ideal, as it coincided with her daughter Liana's 18th birthday party. She asked her oncologist if she could delay the start of treatment, but the answer was a firm 'no'. Twenty-one days later, she had lost all her hair, but that did not stop her from wearing a gorgeous wig and being there for Liana.

For the first three months, Lou had chemotherapy infusions once every three weeks, then the frequency increased to weekly for another three months. She was also prescribed the drug Herceptin.

"I started researching Herceptin and it's like a miracle drug for that type of cancer. It made me feel confident. On one hand they were saying this is a really aggressive cancer and the chances of it coming back are between 30% and 70%, but by having Herceptin, you halve the chances of it coming back so that was great."

I asked Lou if she experienced any side effects from her treatment regime. She was happy to report that she did not feel terribly unwell. Apart from hair loss and constipation, she experienced little nausea and minimal fatigue.

"Maybe I psyched myself into not having side effects because I had just opened a business. It was not a question of, 'Can I have six months off to relax?' Even having two days off every three weeks for treatment was a lot of time off to me. For those two days and the weekend I would generally stay home, but I never let chemotherapy stop me from socialising. I've got photos of me all dressed up at functions."

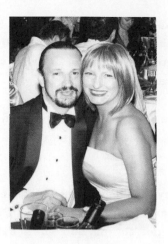

Rob and Lou (in her wig)

Lou was fine until the last three months of weekly chemotherapy. The first time she went for her weekly sessions of chemotherapy and Herceptin, she vomited before the injection. The nurses explained it as anticipatory nausea because, by that point, she had endured so many needles that her veins were difficult to locate and the cannula insertion was painful.

Radiotherapy started after her six months of chemotherapy. Lou had 30 sessions—one each day for six weeks. She is grateful that it did not tire her—she knew that for some, the process was exhausting. The worst effect of the radiotherapy was a feeling that she had a bad case of sunburn, with redness and peeling skin under her breast.

Throughout her treatment, Lou had the incredible support of her parents, family, friends and her husband Rob. Lou describes Rob as a tough talker, always positive and willing to do whatever he could to help her recovery.

One of the biggest lessons Lou learned was to let people help and support her. One evening she came home from work and instead of allowing Rob to serve the wonderful meal he had prepared, Lou picked up the crockpot, not realising that it was still plugged in at the wall. The unexpected pull caused the contents to splash out onto her wrist. She suffered second degree burns.

"I screamed like a maniac and then I had to go to the doctor every single day to have my dressings changed because it was quite bad. It was an act of stupidity, my own fault, but I just can't stay still!"

Lou's daughter Liana was completing her final year of high school. The way Lou's illness affected her children was the hardest thing that she faced.

"I was seeing my oncologist and she asked me how things were going. I started crying and said, 'I'm doing fine but my daughter is not coping and she's driving me insane. We're just fighting all the time.' She suggested we talk to a psychologist which we did, and it was helpful. I was trying to be tough, but she was scared. Cancer has a big impact on the people around you."

I asked Lou what advice she would share with someone who may have just started on their own cancer journey.

"Make sure you have good health professionals. Shed all the people who are negative and just have the positive people around you."

Lou's courageous attitude and her ability to look at her own situation with a broader perspective are two of the key factors that enabled her to deal with her cancer and thrive.

"I didn't lose my breast, I got a good scar in a great position. I thought, 'What if I have to lose my breast? Who cares, it's just a boob. I'm not a topless dancer. I don't have to give up my job as a topless waitress. It could have been worse. From my perspective, I've had a really long and happy life. The things I've done in my lifetime, other people just haven't done. I've travelled a lot, had a good career, had kids. And then I thought, 'I have to stay alive for them.'"

Since treatment, Lou has been 10 years cancer-free. She lives every moment with gusto, travelling the globe and visiting fantastic places. She even had the courage to learn to ride a motorcycle!

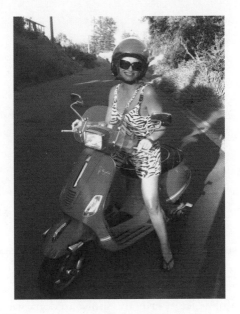

Lou on a vespa

Lou never gave herself the luxury of feeling sorry for herself because she had a family, friends and business that needed her. She kept moving forward and Lou's personal experience has made her a vocal advocate for regular mammograms and early detection. She shares this message by speaking for the national Breast Cancer Foundation and through her participation in the 10,000 Italian Roses Project, a program designed to raise awareness of the importance of mammograms among Italian women.

Lou's law practice has flourished, earning many awards over the years including Businesswoman of the Year.

"I had the sexy disease, the one where money is being pumped into trying to get cures, so I consider myself lucky, rather than unlucky. I look at everything that happened to me as good luck, not bad luck."

4

TIMOTHY

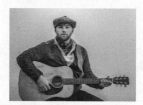

DIAGNOSIS: STAGE 4-B PRIMARY MEDIASTINAL B CELL LYMPHOMA

WHEN YOU LISTEN TO TIMOTHY'S MUSIC, YOU ARE IMMEDIATELY DRAWN in by his beautiful voice, perfectly showcased in songs that speak to your heart. A talented singer-songwriter, Timothy's love of music began as a child singing with his older sister, Clare. It really took hold when he was accepted into St Mary's Cathedral Choir where he sang for four years as head chorister.

At the age of 13, Timothy was the first child to be offered a singing scholarship at a prestigious private school in the Illawarra, a region about an hour south of Sydney.

"I sang my way through high school, taught myself how to play the guitar and started playing more and more. Music was pretty much the only thing I felt I could really do well, so I decided to put all my focus into it."

Timothy's focus earned him a place at the Sydney Conservatorium of Music, Australia's premier tertiary music institution, where he was enrolled in Jazz studies straight out of high school. By the age of 22, he achieved a Bachelor's Degree in Music Studies, (Jazz Vocals) and the question of what to do next. Timing played a big part in Timothy's immediate future plans. Just as Timothy was finishing university, his sister Clare was building a stellar career as an actress having just landed a role as a leading cast member in the U.S. TV show 'Nashville.'

"I just went over there and hung out with Clare as much as I could. There's an incredibly well-established songwriting community in Nashville and I got to meet so many different writers that really opened my own mind to the concept of chasing songwriting as a profession."

Timothy loved the fertile environment in Nashville and began a cycle of living over there for a month or two at a time, coming home to Australia and playing as many shows as possible to earn cash, then flying back over to the United States to soak up the creative inspiration and to learn from musicians who were having great success.

"That really propelled me towards my next goal which was to write songs for other people, as well as for myself, and to work solely as a songwriter."

Spending so much time in Nashville came at a price. Timothy ran himself ragged in order to fund his overseas trips. Timothy found himself playing at two weddings most weekends, as well as up to four pub (hotel/bar) shows during the week. He was happy to be earning money doing what he loved, but it was tough on his voice and his body.

"Playing consistently in pubs is one of the hardest jobs I have ever done as a musician. I was doing five or six gigs a week, would sometimes drive for up to eight hours, then had to set up a PA system and punish my voice for a further three hours singing Cold Chisel and Daryl Braithwaite songs until the bar closed—on most occasions at around 1am."

For three years, Timothy followed this chaotic lifestyle. He wrote and released a few EPs (Extended Play — a short album with four to six songs) and his music was attracting interest from record labels. Timothy was making some great connections and his career was starting to gather momentum.

In mid-2015, when Timothy was 25, a festival performance in Perisher Valley (a popular ski region in Australia) sparked off a strange series of events that led to his timely cancer diagnosis.

Early in the morning after the festival, Timothy was racing off to his fiancé's sister's wedding at Kangaroo Valley, a five-hour drive from Perisher Valley. He started heading north along the main road and just five minutes into his journey, without warning, a car pulled out of a side street right in the front of him and the two vehicles collided.

The airbags deployed and broke Timothy's glasses in two, sending both halves flying to either side of the car. The impact also forced his leg into the drivers' door, straining a ligament in his knee. The car was totalled. It is a miracle that he was able to literally walk away from the crash.

Fortunately, the other driver was not seriously injured either. Within seconds, a highway patrol car was at the scene to assist. The officer had encountered car trouble and stopped his vehicle just moments before the accident, placing him in the right place to witness the incident. The three of them reached for their phones to call for help, but given their remote location, none of them had any cell phone reception.

They were lucky that it was the first day of ski season. A steady stream of cars was heading up the mountain. One car stopped, a woman jumped out and she began running toward the tangle of metal that was Timothy's vehicle.

Unbelievably, she was a family friend from his small home town. She had recognised the car from a distance. Out of everyone at the scene, she was the only one with cell phone reception and she kindly made the calls to friends and family to inform them of what had happened and to reassure them that Timothy was okay.

The next piece of good luck came in the form of Noel, the bass player with whom Timothy had performed the night before. Unbeknownst to Timothy, Noel had been booked to play at the very same wedding that Timothy was trying reach. After discovering what had happened, Noel and the rest of Timothy's band came to the rescue. They finally made it to the wedding just in time for the reception, where Timothy performed his duty as MC for the evening.

Before being cleared to go to the wedding, Timothy had to attend the local hospital to have his injuries checked and to also undertake the mandatory tests required after a car accident. He can still remember this very clearly.

"I had this particularly anxious moment when I was sitting on the hospital bed being examined, thinking, 'They're going to find something else. Something terrifying.' As it turned out, they didn't find anything unusual that day, but I remember that exact moment like a snapshot in my mind and it has stuck with me ever since."

Perhaps it was foreboding of what was to come, or maybe it was Timothy's body communicating to him. Many cancer survivors say that they instinctively knew something was wrong before their diagnosis.

The accident did not slow Timothy down. He was travelling more than ever before. Timothy's fiancé, Christina, was studying to be a doctor at the time. She took up a placement at Lismore Base Hospital, a long ten-hour drive or a short flight away from their home in the Illawarra. Timothy was commuting back and forth at least once a week to see her, on top of his extensive travel around the country for his shows.

Keeping up with such a hectic schedule took its toll. Timothy noticed that he was always very tired, that his back was constantly sore and that he was losing a considerable amount of weight. In the six months following his accident, Timothy lost 20 kg (44 lb). He attributed this to both his increased travel and exercise schedule, thinking nothing more of it.

Timothy remembers playing a show at Café Lounge in Sydney's Surry Hills where a very vocal audience member was enthusiastically enjoying his set. His new fan introduced himself after the show as Reuben. He then told Timothy that he was in town for a few nights playing with singer, Sam Smith and asked whether he would like to come along to a show. Timothy was thrilled, it was too good of an opportunity to pass up. He was, however, also due back in Lismore to help Christina move south for the summer break.

To fit everything into his schedule, he flew north to help pack up her house, flew back to Sydney for Sam Smith's concert, then flew north once again the next day to accompany Christina back on the long drive home. Between travel, exercise, performing and recording, to say Timothy's life was manic would be a gross understatement.

The first sign that something was seriously wrong came when he was crossing a main road in Byron Bay a few days prior to his final journey south with Christina. He was complaining of a sore back from the long journey when he sneezed, and to everyone's surprise, he collapsed on the ground in the middle of the road. After being helped to his feet by a few passers-by, he went straight to a GP who prescribed pain medication.

"To me, all of my symptoms were explainable. I was travelling so much, I thought, 'Of course I'm tired.'"

Timothy continued his busy schedule and his symptoms got worse; he began to experience drenching night sweats, insurmountable lethargy, and further weight loss. Despite these obvious signs, going to the doctor was not a priority for him. Throughout his entire life, Timothy had rarely been unwell enough to warrant a visit to the doctor. He explained to me that his family did not have a particularly strong culture of seeing medical professionals. Past experiences were far from therapeutic, to say the least, stemming from Clare's battle with cancer as a child.

When Clare was four years old, after weeks of unexplainable symptoms, she was diagnosed with Wilm's Tumour, also known as nephroblastoma, a childhood kidney cancer. Their mother, Kathleen, realised that something was wrong with Clare and took her to their local GP. Kathleen was told that she was delusional, there was nothing wrong with her daughter, and that she should try to get more sleep. Kathleen persisted and eventually took Clare to the emergency department at a nearby hospital where a football-sized tumour was found in Clare's abdomen. Doctors gave her two weeks to live. Thankfully, Clare triumphed due to experimental chemotherapy but the dismissive attitude of the doctors at Kathleen's initial concern led to a significant distrust of medical professionals that was passed down to the next generation.

Timothy's back pain was getting worse, so he decided to see a chiropractor. On his first visit, the chiropractor explained that she was going to do a simple adjustment that could feel abrupt, but should not involve any pain.

"When she performed that adjustment, I felt a kind of excruciating pain that I had never felt before. That was the first and only time I have ever uncontrollably screamed out in pain. She got such a fright."

It was just before Christmas of 2015 that, after Christina's persistent requests, Timothy finally went to see a doctor. He was sent for blood tests to investigate his symptoms further, as well as a chest CT scan to rule out fractures from the car accident months earlier.

On the day that Timothy's results came in, he was preparing for the annual yuletide tradition of recording Christmas songs together with family and friends. The recording was made each year and sent out to grandparents and other family members. About half an hour before everyone was due to arrive, Timothy's medical practice phoned and asked him to come in immediately.

His usual doctor was not working that day, however the receptionist insisted. Timothy and Christina had no idea why the request was so urgent but given that the practice was only a few minutes up the road, they went straight away.

"Christina and I showed up and were called into a room with an unfamiliar doctor. Realising the nature of the conversation we were about to have, the doctor came right out and said it was either lymphoma, myeloma or testicular cancer. We were both completely stunned. It was like a weird twilight zone of disbelief. Not disbelief in the sense that this can't be happening, or it's insane, or a place of denial. It was more like, 'That just happened.' I was soaking it in trying to process the information."

As they left the practice, Christina's sister, Kate, was driving past. She stopped and ran over to them, oblivious and excited to begin their night of recording. Timothy was lost for words, so Christina handed Kate, also a doctor, the report from Timothy's CT scan. Large central mass, lymph node and bony involvement, pericardial and pleural effusions…the words swam before her eyes. Kate asked pleadingly, whether there was a mistake. This couldn't actually be Timothy's body housing this strange, sinister invasion, could it? The three of them stood on the sidewalk in disbelief. At that moment, more of Christina's family arrived and stopped to greet them.

"I can't even remember what we said to them in that moment. It was such a blur."

There was no Christmas album that year. They broke the news to their friends who were waiting eagerly at their house. The recording session was cancelled and they all went out for a sombre dinner, sharing a meal and commiserations. Timothy and Christina then drove down to Timothy's family home to deliver the news in person to his parents and via telephone to Clare.

Wasting no time at all, the next day, Timothy had a biopsy taken from his rib, a bone scan, bone marrow biopsy and PET scan. Timothy remembers seeing the PET scan of his body 'lit up like a Christmas tree' as he felt the gentle hand of his oncologist on his knee and heard, "It's a bit more extensive than we thought, mate."

Although Timothy's medical team wanted to start treatment immediately, there were some unavoidable delays due to the approaching Christmas period. There were also some puzzling features about his biopsy. Pathologists were still determining exactly which type of cancer Timothy had. This meant that he was able to be discharged for a few days over Christmas, under the strict proviso that he return if anything adverse happened.

Over the next few days, Christina began to notice some swelling in one of Timothy's arms. She insisted on taking him to emergency.

"I refused to go for the longest time and then ended up having to go because I just felt so sick and awful by Boxing

Day. I eventually just handed it over to Christina and the rest of my family and I said that I needed to go. My stubbornness got a huge lesson there."

Timothy was readmitted to hospital via emergency the day after Christmas. Although his presenting complaint was swelling in his left arm, which by now was red, tender and twice its size, the emergency doctor admitted him to the oncology ward without investigating further, stating that there was "no appreciable difference" between his left and right arm. The swelling increased. Christina pushed for the doctors to take an ultrasound of his arm, but the doctors were hesitant; they did not want to upset the specialist's treatment plan while he was away on holidays. Christina persisted, and after asking four different doctors, the ultrasound was finally conducted. It showed a blood clot from Timothy's wrist all the way to his neck, just below his ear. They estimated that had it been left for just a few more days, he would probably have had a heart attack.

In the days following, after much debate between specialists, he was diagnosed with Stage 4-B Primary Mediastinal B Cell Lymphoma.

Timothy's emergency admission became a month-long stay to confirm his diagnosis, prepare his six-month treatment schedule and complete the first round of chemotherapy. Once discharged, he became an outpatient, with chemotherapy treatment administered through a PICC line in his arm.

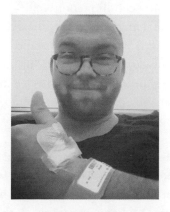

Timothy in treatment

Every three weeks he would attend the Cancer Day Care Clinic at Wollongong Hospital, where nurses would connect a battery-operated pump that would slowly release a concoction of chemotherapy drugs over 96 hours. He would then return to have the pump disconnected and undergo further intravenous infusions and chemotherapy delivered directly into his central nervous system via lumbar puncture. Timothy estimates he endured a total of 800 hours of chemotherapy.

One of the most trying days occurred about halfway through the treatment process. Timothy's medical team decided to harvest his stem cells in the event that they needed to use them later on in his therapy.

The preferred method of collection requires an aphaeresis machine connected to cannulas inserted into both arms, one allowing blood to go into the machine to be separated into different parts, and the other to allow processed blood to be returned to the patient. After multiple unsuccessful attempts to find a vein in Timothy's arm, the medical staff used ultrasound equipment and finally achieved successful placement of the cannula. They switched on the machine only to discover that Timothy's veins could not handle the pressure required for the machine to work.

The alternative plan was to install a vascular catheter to collect blood via the femoral artery in Timothy's groin. The procedure worked flawlessly. Once finished, they removed the catheter and he was instructed to lie still for at least two hours until the incision site became stable, after which he would be able to leave. Timothy dutifully lay still while his Dad stood by to keep him company.

After three hours of lying still, just to be safe, he was given the all clear from the nurses and attempted to stand up from the bed. The moment he put downward pressure on his legs, the catheter site exploded, and blood began to flow down his leg and all over the floor.

Timothy's Dad ran out of the room to find a nurse and a whole team of them came rushing in to help.

"I remember it feeling so bizarre—sitting in a hospital bed as a 26-year old, with nurses who were basically my age, plugging the vein in my groin with their hands to stop me from bleeding out, to keep me alive. I thought to myself,

'This is not a situation people find themselves in during their day-to-day life.' It was so surreal."

As preventative care to reduce the risk of any further blood clots during his treatment, he had to inject Clexane twice daily for six months. The combination of all these treatments proved successful and after just three rounds of treatment, his PET scan showed minimal activity, meaning that all of the tumours that riddled his body just months earlier were gone and that he had technically entered remission. It was under his specialists' recommendation that Timothy completed the full course of his chemotherapy regime which meant undergoing another three rounds of intense treatment.

Around this same time, Clare planned to come back to Australia, after having to return to the U.S. due to work commitments for most of Timothy's treatment. Upon her return, Clare embarked on her first Australian tour and asked Timothy to open all of her shows nationally, health permitting. He jumped at the offer. Timothy scheduled his weekly dressing changes and his final chemotherapy round to work in with the tour schedule, flying back to Wollongong for treatment, then meeting his sister at the next performance venue. Since treatment, he has noticed a change in his mental attitude to many things, and in particular, how he feels when he is on stage.

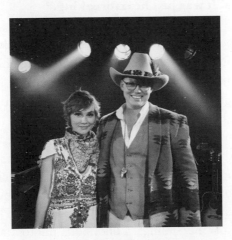

Clare and Timothy on tour

"I used to get awful stage anxiety, particularly getting incredibly nervous about forgetting words and chords and that sort of thing. Now, it doesn't seem to matter. I can just play the songs and I know they are going to have meaning to a lot of people and the anxiety just isn't there anymore. It's good in terms of self-preservation and being able to do your job really well because there are no distractions, no butterflies, no anxiety, none of that."

Timothy had another PET scan six months after being given the all clear. To his and his family's dismay, the scan found inconclusive chemical activity on his sternum, his rib and in the lining of his heart. This sparked the need for further investigation to check if the cancer had returned. Timothy had heart surgery and multiple biopsies taken from the two other sites—thankfully, all came back negative.

That was about 18 months ago now, and Timothy has been doing very well since. I asked him what he felt was the hardest part of his journey and he immediately responded that it was telling his Mum.

"The hardest part of everything that I went through was seeing how my illness affected other people. I think one of the hardest things for me was having to tell Mum. To see her reaction. It was just heartbreaking."

From a support point of view, Timothy is eternally grateful for the world-class hospital care he received and the incredible support of his friends and family. Christina was unwavering in her support throughout the entire experience. Being a doctor in training, she could explain all of the complicated medical jargon in lay terms, when needed. She made sure that Timothy and his family felt supported in every aspect of day-to-day life.

Clare honoured her brother in an incredibly special way with the release of her song "Love Steps In" written by her husband Brandon Robert Young and close friend, Justin Halpin. The music video features photos of the siblings' childhood, photos taken throughout both his treatment and hers as a child. It also contains clips of highlights in Timothy's life, including his invitation to join Clare on stage to perform at the prestigious Grand Ole Opry in Nashville, Tennessee.

"It's funny when you are in those extreme situations. You really find out who your people are, especially when you're laid up in hospital for a month."

In 2017, Timothy was asked to be a Cancer Council NSW Ambassador for their hallmark fundraising day, Daffodil Day. He considered it a great privilege and used his musical talents to write a song for them called "For Someone I Know." The song is dedicated to all of those who supported him, and all the caregivers and supporters helping someone else through their cancer journey.

Timothy is now looking at his priorities and is focussed on continuing his music career. One of the frustrations he faces is that now that his treatment is finished, and the physical signs of cancer are less obvious, there is the expectation for him to just pick up and get on with his life as if nothing happened. He shared with me the challenge of living in a world where people have a short attention span.

"The industry moves on so quickly that after everything that has happened, at times, it can feel really disabling. People give you their best wishes, but as soon as there's no physical sign of sickness any more, it feels as if many forget everything that's happened and everything you're still working through. I don't blame them at all for moving on. I think given the 24-hour news cycle we now live in and the constant stream of social media posts, it's unavoidable. And no one wants to dwell on the past. Though I think most of it is an internal pressure from myself to get back to a state of being that feels familiar to the time that was before cancer. Everything has changed so much however, that it's almost irrelevant to make any comparison. These are all lessons I'm still learning."

For Timothy, the physical side of treating cancer was in some ways easier than dealing with life after treatment had finished. He has found that the primary key to helping him maintain a good mental attitude is predominantly exercise. Purchasing a Fitbit has helped him to set goals and quantify his progress, providing great motivation for recovery.

"I found that exercise was the biggest catalyst in changing my own mental health. I've even noticed a seriously definable pattern where, when I don't exercise for a few weeks, my thoughts tend to lean toward constant negativity, no matter what the situation. It's fascinating."

With music still being the strongest force in his life, Timothy is rebuilding his physical strength and performing regularly. He continues to write amazing songs. His story is about hard work, good luck and an incredibly loving family. These are the things that will support him in whatever is to come.

"When you come so close to not being here, you ruminate on everything that you want to get done in your life. It changes you completely. You have a whole new perspective on everything. It gives you so much fire and determination in your day-to-day life, as well as an incredible amount of understanding and compassion for those around you. And there are so many scars to show for it, but after everything, it's all for the better. I wouldn't change one thing."

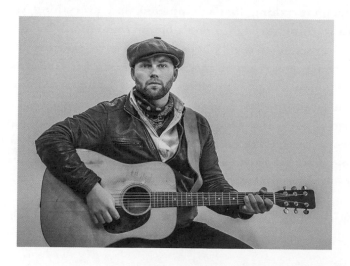

5

VI

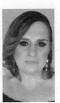

Diagnosis: Burkitt's Non-Hodgkin's Lymphoma

Positive. Strong. Determined. Mentally tough. These are words that flame through my mind as I think of the human dynamo that is Vi. An extraordinary woman of immense courage and tenacity, Vi faced the battle of her life and triumphed.

Vi has risen through the ranks of the banking industry over the last 15 years and today is one of the ANZ's most respected Business Banking Managers. She is a woman absolutely committed to her job and her customers; hardworking, focussed and goal driven.

For Vi, turning 40 marked the beginning of a series of life-changing events. She had suffered an iron deficiency for many years and was bleeding constantly. This condition led to a hysterectomy that went smoothly and, of course, Vi used the recovery to completely overhaul her wellbeing. She lost weight, trained hard and was at her peak fitness level: "a brand new me."

In December 2014, a couple of years later, Vi was experiencing a stressful time at work when she began having extreme pain in the right side of her jaw.

"When it would hit me, I felt like getting myself and knocking myself out! That's how severe it was."

She tried all the usual pain medication, but nothing worked. Self-diagnosing a problem with her wisdom teeth, Vi went to her dentist. He asked her to get X-rays because he could not see a problem. These turned out to be poor quality, and Vi's dentist requested that she obtain more advanced 3D X-rays. By the time she returned with the new X-rays, it was about a week later, and Vi had started developing additional symptoms. Her belly was beginning to bloat, and her jaw pain had become excruciating.

Still unable to see any problem, the dentist sent Vi to an orthopaedic specialist who ordered an MRI. At this stage, Vi was still completely sure it was a dental issue and she imagined that all the pain medication was ruining her stomach lining. The specialist would not give her nerve blocking injections until he saw the MRI, and instead prescribed her with the narcotic, Endone, which made her so ill that she swears she will never take it again.

"I went to get my MRI, and just being in that thing, lying down, you can imagine it. Nobody could tell me what was happening. I thought I may as well just die, there's got to be a better way of living."

At that point, Vi thought she ought to see her GP about her stomach. An X-ray and ultrasound of the area revealed nothing, so he suggested it was constipation, and sent her to get a CT scan. By the time she reached the clinic for the scan, she could no longer fit into her normal clothes and the sonographer asked if she was pregnant. No one had advised that she needed to fast before the scan and so as it was a Friday, the test had to be postponed until the following Monday.

By this stage, Vi was not sleeping: she could not drink water, she looked like she was ready to give birth, she was still in agony and yet she made the huge effort to attend a friend's 40th birthday party the next day. Her husband, Tony was becoming very worried. When Vi arrived at the party, her friend took one look at her and said, "What the hell are you doing here? You should go straight to emergency." Vi replied, "I couldn't disappoint you." Tony made the decision for Vi and they drove straight to hospital.

They walked in, and, seeing so many people waiting, Vi decided that she felt alright and wanted to go home. The next morning, she woke up struggling to breathe, so Tony called an ambulance.

I was stunned to hear that the period from Vi's initial jaw pain through to her arrival at hospital was a mere two weeks. During that time, she had continued going to work every day.

"In between customers, I was going and lying down in the conference room, going behind the chairs and having a nap and then getting back up. Seriously, what was I thinking?"

Vi was fitted with an IV drip and sent for an immediate CT scan and PET scan. These tests revealed a large amount of fluid in her stomach and around both lungs. The medical team took a biopsy of the fluid, and then inserted drains. A total of 10 litres of fluid was removed from her body.

Tests on the fluid finally provided some answers. Vi was diagnosed with Burkitt's Lymphoma, the fastest growing cancer known today. It is associated with impaired immunity and only accounts for 1% of adult lymphoma cases, but up to 30% of child Non-Hodgkin's lymphoma.

Vi's haematologist explained, "There's something here and it's serious, very serious. To put it in perspective, had you not come in today, you would have been dead by Christmas."

The date was 14 December. The fact that she could have been just 11 days from death was a shocking thought for Vi to process. She was admitted to hospital and started on chemotherapy immediately.

"Between my diagnosis and my first chemo treatment, I didn't have time to think. I knew there was only one way forward. I was going to fight this with all my strength and being."

In this moment of crisis, Vi drew on her inner strength to determine her next course of action. Once Vi had her diagnosis, once she knew what she was up against, as with everything else in her life, she focussed 100% of her actions and willpower to getting through treatment and creating the best opportunity for survival.

"I remember telling myself, 'You are stronger than you believe you are.' I know it's scary and we wouldn't be human if we didn't ponder on those negative thoughts running through our mind."

Treatment involved having a PICC line installed in a vein above the bend of her elbow to administer chemotherapy and other medication. This stayed in place for the duration of her treatment. On her second day in hospital, Vi's doctor explained that the other part of her treatment would involve lumbar punctures. Also known as spinal taps, this procedure involves lying very still whilst a needle is inserted into the spinal canal.

This is terrifying enough by anyone's standards, but Vi is petrified of needles; she has a serious phobia of them.

"My joke with the doctors and nurses was that when they asked if I had any allergies, I would say, 'Yes, I'm allergic to needles.'"

Vi's doctor explained that some of the chemotherapy had to be administered this way so that it would not affect her stem cells. He held the consent form for her to sign, and Vi remembers him saying that she was brave even though she was an emotional wreck, crying like a baby and wiping her eyes whilst signing the form.

"I didn't have a choice. I needed to get through this as I wanted to live and be around for my family. This would not be my undoing."

The visit to emergency turned into a long three month stay in hospital. She had chemotherapy every day, and over the course of that 90-day period, she had eight lumbar punctures.

"I would shake. I shook like a leaf when the lumbar

puncture procedure was being done. I'm a strong person, but that would destroy me. They gave me tablets to calm me down, but nothing worked. I always made sure I had someone there to just hold my hand and I kept telling myself this is only temporary, breathe, and it will be over before you know it."

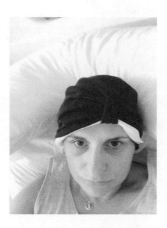

Vi during treatment

Vi has a wonderfully supportive family. Her mother, "a rock," a gentle, caring person, was with Vi when the doctor gave his diagnosis. As soon as she heard the news, her Mum started crying. Vi used all her strength to hold it together until the doctor left the room.

Never one to hold back from her truth, Vi asked her mother if she could keep it together. She could not deal with seeing her mother upset and worrying about her when she needed to concentrate all her energy on fighting for her life.

"I said to Mum, 'I need your support. I can't do this by myself. I cannot have you crying or being negative. Can you promise me that?' I had to say that because I knew that she would have killed me, seriously, watching her crying all the time would have put me in a place I couldn't afford to be in. I couldn't afford to be around negativity, like I'm dying. I didn't want people to look at me and feel sorry for me. I didn't want their pity."

Her Mum was amazing and came in every day trying to make Vi laugh. She remembers having this conversation with her Mum:

> Mum: *"I wish I was in your shoes, if God is going to take anyone,*
> *I want Him to take me."*
> Vi: *"He chose me because He knows I can overcome it."*
> Mum: *"Why do you say that?"*
> Vi: *"Because you know what you're like, you have a headache and*
> *you're dying."*
> Mum: *"You know what, you're probably right."*

Vi admits Tony was a "mess" struggling with his own feelings and concern for his wife, but also having to look after their sons, take care of their home, and still go to work. He bravely talked to the whole family about Vi's wishes for positive support, and on many days, she had 20 encouraging people in her room at once. Even work colleagues and customers would come to visit. Vi found that difficult, but she also acknowledged that it was important to let them come in to understand what was happening to her. It helped them to process their emotions. She had so many visitors that they eventually had to put time restrictions on the ward.

"I needed to stay positive...I decided to only surround myself with people who lift me higher. I was going to need it through this journey."

Vi really appreciated the visits by the Leukaemia Foundation support team.

"It was good to talk to a third party. I had to be cautious with what I said to my family. I didn't want them to panic or to think I was not as strong as I said I was. It was great to get that sounding board every now and again."

The hardest things were the simple things that we take for granted.

"When friends came to visit me straight from work, I was

jealous of the simple things that they could do that I couldn't like being able to walk out of the hospital, going back to their lives while I was stuck in a hospital bed, trying to get there. It really does impact you in one form or another. You just take those little things for granted."

After three months, on 14 March, Vi was discharged and went home. Over the next five months, she gradually recovered. At first, she could not even walk up the stairs and had to be lifted. She needed help with all the little things, like showering and washing her hair. She is so grateful that Tony, her parents and her boys were there to support her —she was never left alone.

Overall, Vi's treatment and recovery took a year. She was pleased to say that her employer was phenomenal, allowing her to work part-time upon her return. Vi also had the advantage of financial security: she had plenty of sick leave and income protection insurance in place.

Vi's journey had a major impact on her family. Her younger son had just finished his final year of high school and it was a difficult time for both of her sons. Vi was brave and open, about her illness but the boys tell her that they were so scared of losing her. Now, Vi has stopped just saying her family is her first priority, she designs her life that way.

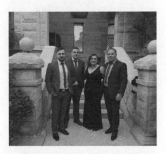

Vi with her sons and husband, Tony

"I used to say family first, work second, but it wasn't. The way I treated my family...I wouldn't even treat my colleagues like that. I'd walk in, always grumpy. I just took them for granted. Now they are number one."

Nine months after her treatment, Vi's CT scan was completely clear. Burkitt's Lymphoma is extremely aggressive, but it is also reactive with the right treatment. Now she only needs annual check-ups and at present, her blood work is perfect. Vi's intentions are to stay well by eating healthy food, using organic products, going to personal training, physiotherapy and whatever else she needs so she can move.

Vi lives by the life motto of treating others as you would like to be treated yourself. Her mother used to tell her to always be kind to everyone including herself because you do not know what burden some people carry on their shoulders. This is not just something that Vi believes, it is something she puts into action daily with small acts of kindness, whether it is paying for someone's groceries, fundraising for causes, giving her time, or simply showing gratitude.

Upon her discharge from hospital, Vi left a letter for the next person who would occupy her bed. It was her way of "paying it forward." The letter contained practical tips, plus some wise advice:

"Believe in yourself, be strong even when you think you can't. I know you can, we are stronger than we give ourselves credit for. It was tough, but I was tougher."

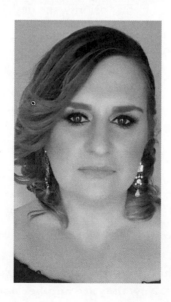

RYAN

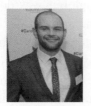

DIAGNOSIS: NEUROENDOCRINE TUMOUR AND BOWEL CANCER

Ryan is one of the most positive young men I have had the honour to meet. Physically fit and determined, he possesses the mental toughness and positive attitude of an elite athlete.

I was excited to meet Ryan together with his fiancé Nicky, a beautiful woman with a sensitive and caring soul. They are a wonderfully complementary couple, together now for 10 years, before and throughout Ryan's cancer diagnosis.

Ryan was just 24 years old when he noticed a few odd symptoms that were totally uncharacteristic. He is typically competitive and goal oriented in everything he does. Whether it is work or his chosen sports of cricket and soccer, Ryan always pushes himself to perform well.

Toward the end of 2012, during the busy period leading up to Christmas, Ryan found he was lacking energy and struggling at work. As a truck driver, he was fearless and would strive to be the best at his job. It was concerning that he was getting slower and slower. He wondered if it was just a temporary slump, but his condition did not improve, and eventually he reached the stage where he could barely finish a day's work.

Ryan also found he was exhausted after bowling a few overs playing competitive cricket. Nicky recalls that he was sometimes so tired that he would almost fall asleep while eating dinner! They realised that something must be wrong and went to see a GP who thought Ryan looked a bit pale and suggested that he was anaemic. The doctor took a blood sample for testing to investigate further.

When the couple returned for the results, the doctor admitted he was surprised that Ryan was still walking around. The blood count revealed that Ryan's haemoglobin was down to 68, the equivalent of living with only half the usual amount of blood in his entire body.

How was the blood loss occurring? An ultrasound showed a lesion in his bowel. The tumour had grown so large that it had ripped a hole in his transverse colon and he was bleeding through the tear. He was haemorrhaging so badly that doctors estimated that another 30 days without treatment would have killed him.

The diagnosis came back as a Grade 3 Neuroendocrine Tumour from his transverse colon to his smaller abdominal cavity. He also had carcinoma in that area. Within a week, Ryan was booked in for surgery.

Nicky recalls how she felt on the day of Ryan's diagnosis:

"I remember waiting, waiting, waiting, and waiting. This team of eight people eventually came to the door and my heart dropped. As soon as they said the diagnosis, I just burst out crying. I literally bawled my eyes out."

Ryan had a completely different immediate reaction:

"Am I going to live or die? What's my chance of survival? Good? Okay, then what's the game plan? What do we do now? It was like on the sporting field, what do we have to do to win? Obviously in this situation, I didn't know so I said to the doctor, 'You're the captain, tell me what we need to do.'"

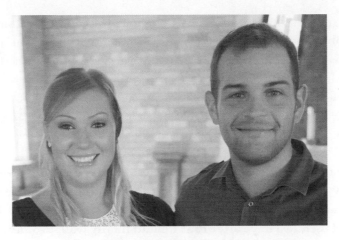

Nicky and Ryan

Everyone reacts differently in times of crisis and there is no right or wrong reaction to a cancer diagnosis. People's responses vary and the emotional state of every patient, family member, friend or carer is totally and absolutely valid and likely to have been formed from a combination of their own personality and life experiences.

Nicky had previously encountered cancer when her Dad was diagnosed in early 2012 and this provided her with some context. The difference was that her Dad had led a fairly unhealthy lifestyle and though she was upset, Nicky was not completely surprised. In contrast, Ryan was young, athletic and consciously chose a healthy diet. He had never, at any time in his life, drunk alcohol or smoked, therefore his diagnosis was a complete shock to both Nicky and Ryan.

From the moment Ryan heard that his prognosis was good, all he wanted to know was what he had to do to defeat the cancer. He was blessed to have one of the country's leading specialists in the field of endocrinology who also happened to be a school-peer of Ryan's step-grandfather's daughter. She was almost like an extended member of the family. Ryan developed a great trust in her judgement.

Ryan's surgery went very well as a result of his healthy lifestyle. His surgeons were happy with the results and commented that his liver and kidneys were textbook examples of how everyone's organs should look, but rarely do. Ryan came out of surgery hooked up to an IV, catheter, bile drain and feeding tube that was installed in his neck.

Ryan's determined attitude throughout his cancer treatment was admirable, and upon hearing his story, I honestly believe that it played a major role in the swiftness of his recovery. Each day he set himself small challenges to keep his recovery moving in a forward direction. One of his first goals was to get up and walk. The medical staff informed him that this was usually possible around the seven-day mark. This information gave Ryan a target to beat.

"It took me four days before I could stand up. I tried every day those first four days, but me being so competitive, I wanted to get up now! It took four days to get on my feet and then two days after that I could finally walk around."

Ryan continued to extend his challenges. He got to the stage where the nurses would do his observations at 6am, and then he would put on his headphones, tune out the environment and walk the whole floor. The following week he did two laps, then three, and then four. Whenever the nurses would see him they would ask, "How many today?"

The other goal he had to achieve in order to get back to regular eating was a clear bile bag. Each day he would send Nicky a photo of his bag, pointing out that it was becoming clearer and clearer. After 23 days, he resumed normal eating and on day 27, he was discharged.

Nicky did her best to visit Ryan every day, but her job involved long hours; she often did not finish work until 8pm. She was totally exhausted and would visit most days, but sometimes needed some alone time. For family and support people, the journey can be as difficult as the trauma experienced by their loved one. Not only do they have to continue their daily lives, but on top of that comes the physical, emotional and time commitment of caring for the patient while dealing with their own worry about their progress and prognosis.

Ryan and Nicky had already discussed the logistics of Ryan's recovery once they were informed that it could take up to a year. They were fortunate to have the support of Ryan's parents who invited them to move into their home during this time. Ryan's parents became part of his support team and their generosity alleviated any financial concerns. Ryan's Polish mother was more than happy to assist in the care of her son and his Dad went above and beyond by accompanying Ryan to medical appointments and keeping him company watching Sopranos while Nicky was at work.

Once discharged, Ryan's oncologist insisted they get started with chemotherapy. Due to the dosages required, he was advised to have a Portacath surgically installed. Unfortunately, the medical team had not realised that Ryan was on the blood thinner Clexane. He woke from surgery with blood all over his chest and remembers seeing the whole staff crowding around him. They apologised and re-anaesthetised him, returning him to theatre to fix the problem.

Ryan's chemotherapy regime involved going to oncology every fortnight on a Monday to have a bottle plugged into his Portacath. He would wear it over the following two and a half days as it slowly infused the chemotherapy drug into his system. Then on the Wednesday afternoon, he would go back to have it removed. This went on for 12 cycles over a six-month period.

Ryan handled the chemotherapy quite well, and naturally asked what activity he was limited to on treatment days, and what he could do on the other days. He was advised to take it easy for at least one day after the treatment, and then to resume light activity. In particular, he had to stay out of the sun because the drug they were using removed the melanin from his skin. Ryan's standard dress when exiting the house became a shirt with long sleeves and a big hat.

As his regular work was physical, he was not allowed to resume that until after the chemotherapy. In the meantime, he needed to find something to keep him occupied.

"Having a little bit of ADD, I had to do something meaningful. I played cricket for the Lake Illawarra Club, and I had heard of another club in Kiama that did the whole stats of their cricket club. Six months is a long time to do nothing, so this made me feel like I was doing something, I wasn't just wasting time."

Ryan walked to the library every day for the entire six months and searched through the microfilm to compile his club's entire statistical history from 1946 to today. This task gave him purpose during that time and a great sense achievement.

In between Ryan's final two chemotherapy treatments, his cricket club's third-grade team needed an extra player. Ryan usually played first grade, but thought he could fill the position and asked his doctor if it would be okay. She agreed as long as he promised not to get hit.

"So, I played the semi-final and grand final in between chemo, which was good. It was a bit of a win that I could go back and play cricket that year, I didn't miss everything. Small steps, small wins."

Ryan returned to work just a month after finishing chemotherapy. He had only needed nine months off work to regain a full level of functioning. Ryan's doctor was so impressed that she included him as a case study in her research. His type of cancer was usually only found in individuals within the forty to sixty-year old age group and not those in their twenties. Ryan's age and excellent recovery made him a particularly interesting case.

Ryan continued with three monthly check-ups due to the severity of his case. In 2015, three years later, a growth showed up in his liver. They monitored it over the following months, and eventually his surgeon decided to remove it based on the formation, size and movement of the mass. Upon testing, the mass was not cancerous and though it involved another three and a half months off work, Ryan does not regret having it removed.

Right now, his medical team is keeping a close watch on any developments. Ryan was happy to tell me that his check-ups are now every six months.

I asked Ryan what he has learned throughout his journey. One of the main things was that it has made him really value the close relationships in his life.

"I appreciate friends and family. Even if you just go to your friend's house for an evening, that sort of good close time can so easily be taken away. You can get so much out of something so simple as having a laugh with people."

Throughout his journey, Ryan appreciated being treated normally. He did not want to feel alienated and found that some people did treat him differently once they knew he had cancer. One of the things that helped was being kept in the loop with his cricket team, even though he was not playing. Being part of the group messaging made him feel like himself, connected and still part of the team.

Ryan and Nicky are now looking toward their future together. Ryan was hesitant to propose to Nicky, not wanting her to feel tied down if he got sick again. His thinking was that it was not fair on her. I asked Nicky how she felt about that and she did not miss a beat, saying, "So next February we'll get married, on our 10-year anniversary."

They have made the decision not to have children due to the multiple cases of cancer in their families. Ryan's father passed from brain cancer last year and this had a big impact on him.

"To see what my Dad went through with me, twice, I'd hate to feel like I contributed to giving cancer to my child. Some people say you can't live your life like that, but you can live your life knowing you definitely didn't pass it on if there is no child. So, we're going to live a great life together."

Nicky does not feel that she is missing out by not having children:

"All of our friends have kids, and we have two beautiful god-daughters," said Nicky. "We get to do the fun stuff and love on them…and then give them back!"

Ryan and Nicky do have another member in their family—Zel is their adorable fur baby and they are totally besotted!

"You don't go backwards, you just try to get better every day. Sometimes your win might be small, but it is still better than it was yesterday. And to me, that's all it was; just got to keep winning, keep getting better."

7

ANNIE

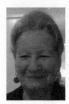

Diagnosis: Cervical Cancer

At just 71 years young, Annie is revelling in her new career as an actress. Spirited, funny and full of enthusiasm, Annie has faced health battles on many fronts, and yet she still forges ahead, determined to enjoy life fully.

Annie's fascinating story begins in the UK. Her father was tailor to King George VI, operating from a prestigious shopfront on London's famous Saville Row while the family home was in Brixton, a South London suburb. As a young child, she spent much of her time playing with neighbourhood friends Helen and Davy, and the three of them would get up to plenty of mischief.

Around 35 years later, Annie's uncle rediscovered a photo of the three friends and gave it to Annie with a smile. He asked if she remembered young Davy Jones because he grew up to become famous singer, songwriter and actor, David Bowie! Her childhood brush with fame was a good omen for Annie who always dreamed of being involved in acting and musicals.

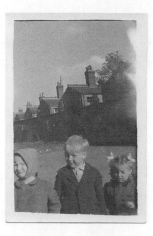

Annie, Davy and Helen

In 1963, her family migrated to New Zealand. Settling into their new life as 'Kiwis' Annie finished her schooling, married and looked forward to creating a family of her own. After two miscarriages, Annie's doctor told her to give up any hope of being a mother as she would never successfully carry a child to full term. This caused a rift between Annie and her husband, and they decided to divorce.

Years later Annie met her second husband and she decided to obtain a second opinion on having a baby. The more I have gotten to know Annie, the more I realise that the concept of "giving up" does not exist for her. Annie went to a different doctor, who advised her to stop taking the contraceptive pill that she had been on since her miscarriages. Within a fortnight, Annie was pregnant!

At age 36, it was a tough pregnancy with complications including gestational diabetes. Annie battled through and gave birth to Cherie, a perfectly healthy little girl.

Annie threw herself into motherhood, and despite various symptoms, she was totally focussed on Cherie and not really paying attention to what was happening to her own body. Niggly conditions such as dry skin, frequent skin infections and weight gain were annoying more than anything, but when her husband pointed out that Annie had not had her period for 18 months, she realised she needed to get checked.

From the symptoms she described, Annie's GP diagnosed early

menopause despite her age of 39. Back in the 1960s, hormone therapy and natural remedies to alleviate menopause symptoms did not exist; the advice from her doctor was to "put up with it and eat less." Years later, Annie would find out that this diagnosis was totally incorrect.

At the time, Annie took the news in her stride and got on with life. The new family moved to Tamworth, a large country town in New South Wales. Annie's husband purchased a funeral business for her to run. She became a funeral director and grew the business into a thriving enterprise. Her passion for helping people soon earned her company a stellar reputation and Annie became a local identity.

When she turned 53, after 17 years with no period, Annie suddenly began bleeding. The first instance occurred when she was visiting family in New Zealand and upon seeing a doctor, she was diagnosed with gastroenteritis and advised that it was nothing serious and would pass. This turned out to be yet another wrong diagnosis.

The condition did not pass. Annie continued bleeding periodically and one morning, she woke up with a bad stomach pain that worsened to the point when she felt like it was going to explode. Moments later a large blood mass just dropped out of her onto the floor.

Annie was rushed to Tamworth Hospital, which was, at the time, too small to handle complicated cases. They admitted her and planned to move her to a larger hospital within a few days.

Upon hearing the news, Annie immediately refused to stay—she needed to perform a funeral service. Despite her serious medical condition, Annie insisted on discharging herself from hospital. She went back to work to take care of her friend's funeral, before returning to readmit herself to hospital.

"More than anything, I'm passionate about helping people."

When she arrived at the John Hunter Hospital in Newcastle, Annie underwent a series of tests which finally provided some answers. The gynaecologist explained that Annie had a 9 cm (3.54 in) tumour growing over her cervix. Cervical cancer is a slow growing cancer, and for the tumour to grow to this size, it had obviously been there for years, most likely since her mistaken early menopause diagnosis.

"When I got cancer, I couldn't believe it! I thought, 'What's God doing to me? Why has he done this?' I struggled really, really hard, because I knew I had to keep running the business no matter what. I'd built up such a good reputation and kept working even while I was lying there dying, because we thought I was going to die, but I just wasn't going to let it happen."

Annie gathered all her strength and willpower to get through the harrowing series of treatments that followed. Her doctor informed her that the tumour could not be removed surgically and would need to be shrunk with chemotherapy, radiation and brachytherapy.

Annie's chemotherapy began immediately at Calvary Mater Hospital, Newcastle, four hours' drive from her home in Tamworth. She remembers it as one of the worst times of her life, living in a hospice next to the hospital so that she could attend daily treatment.

"It was a horrible place. They were all cancer sufferers, all these old, old people. I wasn't old. It smelled of burnt toast. I did not want to be there."

Annie's situation was intolerable: she was living away from her daughter; her parents were in their eighties and living in New Zealand and unable to assist; her in-laws were largely unsupportive; Annie's business was suffering, and her husband could not cope without her. She was utterly alone.

Due to the severity of her case, Annie had Cisplatin chemotherapy administered intravenously for many hours each day for around six months. The environment and the effect of the drug left the usually active and vibrant Annie completely exhausted.

"I had that tiredness that you can't get rid of, and I don't think it ever really goes away."

Unfortunately, the worst was yet to come. Brachytherapy was in its infancy and Annie was used as an experimental case. She consented to the procedure, but even her positive attitude was sorely tested by the procedure. Stage 1 was an operation to insert "skewers" inside her pelvic area. Stage 2 involved being locked in a lead-lined room and laying on a lead bed and mattress for seven days. To enable this, Annie was connected to a colostomy bag, and also had blood transfusions to counteract her low blood count.

After 12 hours on the bed, she felt her mattress deflate. The procedure was stopped, and Annie was sent home. Two weeks later, she had to go through both Stage 1 and 2 again. A few hours into her second attempt, Annie could not believe it when the mattress deflated again! Unwilling to endure any more delays, she decided, with gritted determination, to just lie on that flat mattress and get it over with.

The nurses were afraid to enter the radioactive room and the door was only opened once every 24 hours to deliver Annie's meals for the entire day. As she shared this part of her story, Annie's emotions overwhelmed her. She was lost for words to describe her horrific experience. Is it any wonder Annie is still frightened of hospitals?

Her greatest support during her treatment and recovery was Cherie. On weekends, Cherie would make the long drive to see her Mum. Annie spoke wistfully about the effect her illness and recovery has had on her daughter. I hear both guilt and gratitude in her voice:

"I think the last 18 years have been awful for Cherie, it must have really knocked her about. She's had to do everything for me because my husband left and moved to Newcastle. He just didn't want to deal with it."

Annie was finally released from her "prison camp." She was happy to be going home. It was a difficult time because she suffered from radiation enteritis causing diarrhoea, nausea and vomiting. Annie shrank from clothing size 18 down to size 8. Barely able get out of bed, Annie continued managing her funeral business by phone, until her husband sold it without her knowledge.

"He went absolutely crazy, sold the business and divorced me, but thought he was still married to me. Yeah, it was just horrific."

Annie suddenly found herself divorced, homeless and with no source of income. It is hard to imagine, after suffering such physical and emotional trauma, being able to summon the strength to keep moving forward. Despite her situation, Annie did just that, finding a home and creating a new life for herself.

It took a good two years for Annie to regain health. She was living on a meagre pension when a dear friend had a stroke. The epitome of selflessness, Annie moved in with the elderly lady and became her carer. This continued until her friend went into respite care.

At this time, Annie's ex-husband asked her to come back and live with him. It was five years after their divorce and Cherie had moved into Annie's tiny house. Annie did not want to uproot Cherie again, so she agreed to the arrangement. Soon, however, it became untenable and eventually she removed herself from the debilitating situation and made her way back to Tamworth where she now lives on her own.

Annie has always been interested in the arts, and as a member of both the Tamworth Dramatic and Music Societies, she had performed in a few shows prior to being a funeral director. Upon her return to Tamworth, Annie saw an advertisement in the local newspaper looking for actors and actresses. She phoned the number and was offered a paid role as a featured extra with a speaking part. It was her first foray into the world of movies and she loved it!

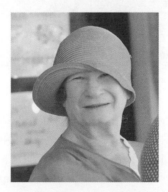

Annie on the set of "Unbroken"

On the day of filming, Annie was a featured extra, appearing right at the beginning of the movie. After her scene, Annie was waiting on a chair for further instructions when, to her surprise, Angelina Jolie came out of a tent and walked directly over to her and started chatting. "You did an excellent job, you look absolutely marvellous," said Angelina.

Annie was so thrilled to be singled out, enjoying a lovely conversation with Angelina for around 10 minutes. Cameras were not allowed, however one of Annie's friends was an official photographer for the local newspaper and he captured a wonderful image of that special moment. The photo was sent around the globe, published in The London Age, Famous Magazine and People Magazine. Since then, Annie has featured in various other videos for the Home Nursing Group and Aged Care Channel.

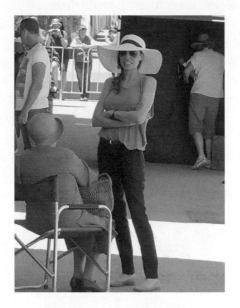

Annie chatting to Angelina Jolie

Annie still lives with the after-effects of her treatment, but she does not let that stop her from embracing life. A fall revealed that her bones were so brittle they had turned to chalk. "They were just floating around in there," she explains. The medical staff told her that they could not operate and that there was nothing they could do to fix the break. Annie was told to "give up living."

That was never an option for this courageous woman. Someone suggested Annie try supplementation, so she started taking glucosamine, magnesium and chromium and, after three years, Annie still uses a walking frame, but she has reduced her morphine medication dose from 40 mg down to 2.5 mg per day. She also believes her diabetes has improved by drinking Tasmanian Blueberry Boost Tea. Amazingly, a recent bone density test showed that her bones are back to normal.

Today, Annie is assisted by the Home Nursing Group who help her with care and medical appointments. She also enjoys the Cancer Aid App which helps her record her journey and access other people's stories.

Nothing stops Annie from enjoying the things she loves. She regularly auditions for acting roles and keeps in touch with the world via social media. She is involved with the Tamworth Music Festival, and attends shows, concerts and musicals with her beautiful daughter Cherie. They have a wonderful relationship and Annie beams with pride when she tells me about Cherie's successful career as a corporate training manager.

Annie is a beautiful soul with an indomitable spirit. Despite being misdiagnosed several times, Annie is not bitter. Told multiple times throughout her life that she should "give up," Annie has refused to be defined by others, making her own choices, changing her circumstances and taking control of her life. To Annie, age is just a number—her best is yet to come.

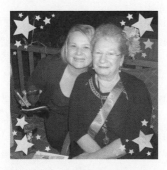

Cherie and Annie at her 70th Birthday

"I don't know why I went through it, but I often think to myself, 'Well I'm glad I did because now I know what it's all about.' My doctor says I'm a miracle, but I just didn't give up."

8

CATUR

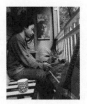

DIAGNOSIS: PSEUDOMYXOMA PERITONEI CANCER

Catur's story cannot be told without Sarah, his partner and soulmate. Together they are the whole package: Catur is the magnetic, spiritual and intuitive musician, while Sarah is a dynamic, articulate and passionate communicator.

The quotes in this story are from Sarah. They provide a unique perspective on the impact that cancer has on those closest to the diagnosed person.

The couple lived in Catur's home country, Indonesia, running their own entertainment company. It was an innovative concept, bringing the joy of African drums and dance to Bali. Catur and Sarah both performed with the many artists they sponsored from Africa, educating in schools and community classes, and entertaining at corporate functions, weddings and gigs at Bali Safari & Marine Park. With bookings seven days a week, and two young boys, Catur and Sarah's life was busy and full.

Catur's first symptoms appeared in 2011 when he started becoming unusually fatigued. Catur and Sarah put it down to their immense workload—they had just expanded their business with two new projects and it seemed like the logical explanation. However, it did become a real concern when his tiredness became more frequent and additional symptoms such as digestive issues began to appear.

As Australian expatriates, they went to the international hospitals in Bali and this was an expensive exercise. Catur visited several hospitals because the diagnoses of irritable bowel syndrome, and the advice of medical professionals to eat on time and to stop eating chilli, were absolutely useless. Catur and Sarah persisted by asking for different types of testing, but no concrete diagnosis was made.

"He was 30 years old. We were young, wild and free. We were running a business that was taking over our lives and we had two young children."

It was now early 2013 and, as they did every year, Catur and Sarah packed down their business and returned home to Australia for their annual two-month break. By this time Catur's tummy had swollen dramatically and Sarah described it to me as the size of her own when she was eight months pregnant!

Sarah made an appointment for Catur with their local Australian GP. The doctor took one look at his distended stomach and, realising that something was seriously wrong, arranged immediate blood tests. Catur was called in for the results that same afternoon: it was cancer, but further testing was required to pinpoint the type and location.

Catur endured three weeks of testing that did not yield a definitive diagnosis—his CT scans showed his organs were clear and an attempt to draw fluid from his stomach was unsuccessful. The next step was a colonoscopy. A strong memory for Sarah is walking beside Catur as he was being wheeled in for this procedure, with the bowel specialist advising her to put Catur's affairs in order because he was betting it was bowel cancer.

Unless you have been in that position, it is impossible to imagine the effect this type of comment has on the patient and their family.

"When you get told you've got cancer, everyone reacts differently. A common reaction is to keep it all to yourself. You don't want anyone to know because it's almost like you

feel contagious. So Catur was very much like that the first month. He didn't want anyone to know. He shut down. And I felt quite isolated, because I felt I needed someone to support me."

Sarah tells me that Catur's grasp of the English language is not great, so at every appointment she would break down the information into plain English. In actual fact, she noticed she tended to sugar-coat her explanations to help him deal with what was happening.

Catur wanted to continue on with life as normal and even performed at a local folk festival in between tests. He was in a state of denial, whereas Sarah was a ball of anxiety with innumerable questions racing around her mind. How was she going to make him understand? What were they facing? What were they up against?

The colonoscopy was clear with no cancer detected in his bowel. By eliminating this as a cause, Catur was sent to St George Hospital in South Sydney to the leading specialists in peritoneal cancer. Due to the urgency of his case, Catur was seen immediately. After another CT scan, they were told that if he walked out of the doctor's rooms that day, Catur's cancer was so advanced that he would be dead in a week.

"We were in a state of disbelief. How can he die in a week? He just performed on stage and boarded a plane and came here and he's still working every day. He's 30 years old and he's just got a big tummy and he's tired. That was our thinking."

It was too much for the couple to process and they decided to go home that day. Within 72 hours, Catur's skin turned grey, he was sleeping all day and could barely swallow a mouthful of food. Sarah called the hospital and was instructed to bring him in straight away. The next day he was on the operating table where they removed six kg (3.3 lb) of tumour in a 13-hour surgery.

Pseudomyxoma Peritonei Cancer is difficult to diagnose as it grows in the walls of organs in the abdominal cavity, such as the stomach lining. For Catur, it started in the stomach lining and then invaded the space around the organs. His cancer grew so large that his organs could not function. His spleen and gallbladder were removed, plus two-thirds of his large bowel as there was secondary bowel cancer on the outside wall of his bowel. The procedure is appropriately nicknamed MOAS, the Mother of All Surgeries.

Catur was given a 50/50 chance of survival and those 13 hours of waiting were some of the hardest for Sarah to bear. She was fortunate that family arranged accommodation at a hotel near the hospital, and the moment she received the call that he was out of surgery and could visit, Sarah scrubbed herself from head to toe because she was frightened about transferring anything that could cause infection.

Catur's recovery was slow. He was fitted with an ileostomy and fed intravenously for the first two weeks. This was followed by two weeks on liquids, then the very gradual introduction of food to get the bowels working again. He was also given Hyperthermic Intraperitoneal Chemotherapy (HIPEC), a concentrated chemotherapy treatment poured directly into the abdominal cavity.

Catur stayed in hospital for over 12 weeks and when he finally came home, it was with some fear and trepidation. Catur still had his drains in and was also required to take an oral chemotherapy treatment called Xeloda, for six months. Responsibility for his medical regime landed squarely on Sarah's shoulders. She had no choice but to become nurse and carer.

"I'm not trained as a nurse, so he was anxious, and I was anxious. It's a huge business for the carer. I developed panic and anxiety attacks."

The Xeloda chemotherapy caused side effects of nausea, vomiting and burnt fingers and toes. It was only after that treatment was completed that Catur started to get back on his feet. He was housebound, physically unable to go anywhere and mentally deflated. When he had his bad days, Sarah would call up his friends to come and play music to him as it would help him feel better.

"It was a relief for me because my heart was breaking, watching him like that. I thought, 'What can I do?' And there was nothing I could do. It's devastating seeing the

**person you love struggle. All you can do is keep supporting
them and just wait."**

It was now April, and the family had expected to be back in Bali,
ready to reopen their business for the start of the season. Instead they
were stuck in Australia with Catur fighting for his life and Sarah
dealing with the very real and practical issue of survival.

**"We were here on our normal two-month holiday, so we had
no funds, nowhere to live. Our business shut down
immediately because we were not there to work it. We had
nothing."**

The one thing the family did have was a wide network of contacts.
As entertainers, Catur and Sarah had helped people and made friends
from all over the world. It was a big step for Sarah to take, but she
knew it was her last option.

**"It was so terrifying to even ask for help. Even though we
had a massive network, we'd never asked for help, ever. It
was almost a pride thing. Your ego goes through many
lessons. So that was a really big thing for me to actually put
it out there publicly."**

Eventually it was Catur's family who told her to go ahead. She
recalls them saying, "Sarah, you are going to have to swallow your
pride. You're going to have to ask for help because you're not able to
support him each day."

While he was still in hospital, through crowdfunding, she had been
able to rent a cheap holiday house near the hospital and her family
took turns coming to the house to babysit so that she could sit by
Catur's bed every day. Sarah had three older children from a previous
relationship and her youngest daughter aged 14, dropped out of school
to look after Catur and Sarah's 13-month-old baby. Sarah's mother,
who was taking care of their seven-year-old son, would come up on
weekends to give them a break.

"When people heard Catur's story, they were devastated. He's a humble man with a beautiful energy about him, and he radiates that like a magnet. People are attracted to him and he is much loved in the community."

Their large network of friends came together to support Catur and his family. A fundraiser held in their local community hall raised $13,000 and that money funded their lives for the 12 months of Catur's recovery. The money raised also helped to purchase a rooftop tent for a seven-week driving holiday in the Australian outback. They drove straight up to Darwin, then back to Uluru.

"We had never done that before…some parts were actually more terrifying than the cancer! We were very disconnected as a family. Our boys had been hiding in their rooms on their iPads because of the relentless vomiting and all the yucky things that kids shouldn't see. That time out in the desert was the best medicine ever because it helped bring our family unit back together."

When they took off on the trip, Catur was still very ill. After a few days on the road, Sarah was worried that they would have to turn back, but she noticed something change in him.

"The challenges of each day, having to set up the tent, made him feel like a man again, that he was still capable. I think that was good medicine for him."

The family returned on a natural high with confidence in their future. They played festivals and felt that no matter what came their way, they would be able to handle it.

Two years on from his diagnosis, Catur was scheduled for a routine stomach bag reversal. With everything going well, the surgeon would reconnect his bowel and he would be rid of the bag. In the lead-up to the operation, Catur was feeling quite anxious. He is very in tune with his body and sensed that the medical team was being evasive. Sarah decided to stay close to the hospital and it was lucky that she did. Two hours into surgery the doctors phoned her to say that Catur was full of cancer again. She was given the option of closing him up and keeping him in hospital to perform the same MOAS surgery again in six to eight weeks, or she could come in and sign the consent form for them to continue on with the MOAS immediately while he was anaesthetised.

Sarah signed the consent form and Catur woke up from his induced coma feeling confused, wondering why he had a ventilator down his throat and all the same drains that he had after the first operation.

"He was absolutely shattered. It was soul-destroying for him. And then we went through the whole thing again."

This time, Catur's physical recovery was faster, but mentally it was much longer and harder to overcome. The doctors suggested intravenous chemotherapy instead of the Xeloda but Catur was reluctant. It was Sarah that talked him into it on the advice of the medical team and it is a decision she regrets. Catur was told that he would have chemotherapy cycles at three-week intervals and that he would likely be sick for five days, and then gradually build up and feel better before the next cycle. The reality was vastly different—he was violently ill for 10 to 20 days each cycle, throwing up continuously. His body was shaking constantly, he was feverish and had an extreme metal taste in his mouth. There was absolutely no quality of life.

While he was receiving the third round, Catur went into anaphylactic shock and pandemonium ensued with medical staff rushing in to revive him. When he can home later that day, Catur said:

"I'm done. I don't want anybody touching me ever again."

This was the point where the couple started to question their medical team. Sarah researched support groups for patients with Catur's type of cancer and could only find one in the USA. She asked lots of questions and was directed to medical reports and studies that showed that there was not one case that was helped by chemotherapy because this type of cancer has a jelly mucous membrane around the cell that chemotherapy cannot penetrate.

Sarah presented this to Catur's medical team and she was told that by law they had to give him a treatment plan. Sarah was obviously upset, replying, "You should have told us, 'These are the facts, make up your own mind.' We just followed what they told us and that put him in more danger than good."

It was a difficult thing for Catur and Sarah to do. The last thing they wanted to do was alienate their medical team, but the lack of transparency made them question the doctor's advice. Not to mention the two clinical errors that occurred during the second operation. Catur's femoral nerve was clamped too long and his legs were paralysed for three months. Worse still, sometime during the surgery he was given an accidental vasectomy and was not informed that it had occurred.

Catur refused any further chemotherapy, and Sarah began investigating alternative therapies. Many friends had sent recommendations about a variety of treatments and, in particular, reports on the efficacy of cannabis oil.

"I wasn't sure if I was doing the right thing or if I was going to hurt him by giving it to him. I wasn't sure if I was going to get into trouble, it was really frightening but we had nothing else to lose."

Within three months of taking cannabis oil, Catur had completely weaned himself off every opioid, painkiller and antidepressant. For the last three years he has treated himself with cannabis oil and the only medication he now takes is aspirin and amoxicillin to compensate for his removed spleen.

Sarah feels that managing his own disease has restored Catur's dignity and confidence. It has given him and his family back their quality of life.

At the end of 2016, the couple was applying for a disability pension and needed a letter from their specialist to support the application. When the letter arrived, it listed Catur as having terminal status, with less than six months to live. The couple were totally baffled. Not once in the past three years had any medical doctor said the word terminal. They had been continuing their life with no knowledge of this prediction on his lifespan. With this new information, Sarah asked Catur what he wanted to do more than anything. Whatever it was, she would make happen. Catur replied:

"I just want to get on a bus and get out of here. I just want to enjoy the rest of my life, however long that is."

Sarah jumped online and reached out to their community again and raised $6,000 online and another $4,000 with a local fundraising event. They found a bus, converted it for their purpose, went through the arduous process of registration and licensing and finally drove off in March 2017 for the trip of a lifetime around Australia.

A local radio station gave them $2,000 in fuel vouchers, and adult wish company, Dreams 2 Live 4, gifted Catur with music equipment so that he could play and perform around the country.

It was a massive community effort and the support continued throughout their entire journey. The first stop was at the Central Coast, about an hour north of Sydney, where the local Indonesian community arranged a fundraiser with more than 100 people. They raised $2,300 and that became their travelling money.

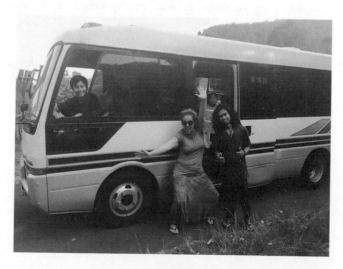

The bus!

Everywhere they went, people were incredible. They earned extra travel money by selling souvenirs online, their music CDs, and through Sarah doing massages. People were reading and following their story on Sarah's blog and Facebook account and would offer their driveways, their homes and their vacant holiday houses for them to stay in.

I asked Sarah how she felt about all the generous support they have received over the past five years.

"It's so strange. I get choked up even now. Our community has gone way beyond. People wanted to help, and they didn't know how. We had people mowing our lawns, babysitting, bringing groceries, cooking. This is something we've learnt, that when people want to help, just accept the help in whatever form they give. A lot of the time all they can do is give money because they might be far away from you or they might even feel confronted. We found that even some close friends found it very confronting and didn't come around for a few months, purely because they just didn't know what to say."

Sarah and I discussed coming to terms with the concept of allowing people to experience the joy of giving by graciously receiving. It is an important lesson they have learnt along the way.

The family travelled across the top of Australia. Catur had his check-up CT scans in Darwin, before they drove the bus down the West Australian coast. Upon their arrival in Perth, Catur received a summons from his medical team saying that they had looked at the scans and he needed to come in urgently for emergency surgery to remove a mass in the front of his abdomen.

Catur stayed awake for 72 hours after receiving the news and eventually said, "no." He had decided to do things his way, and instead of rushing back for surgery, the family went to Indonesia for a month so that Catur could connect with his spiritual leaders and heal.

"I think it brought him into himself. He now understands who he is, where he comes from and where he's going. It

just reinforced the decision not to have medical intervention."

Sarah admits that she struggles with the decision more than Catur because she does not want to lose him. Sarah has to constantly remind herself that it is his body, his decision and even though it is difficult, she knows that she has to make peace with it.

The family plans to go back to Indonesia in July for five months. Catur has a calling and has entered into a spiritual commitment, training every day to become a healer himself. And Sarah and the boys will be there to support him every step of the way.

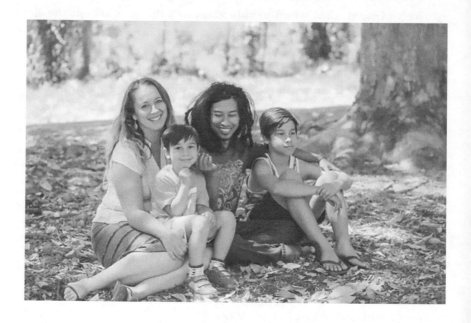

"I'm a big believer that out of every tragedy, there's a gift. As horrible as cancer is, there are so many positives, so many lessons learned. We're not the people we were five years ago. We're actually better at being good people. How can you not? It strips away every layer of ego until you get down to that core self."

9

THIT

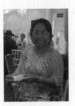

DIAGNOSIS: BREAST CANCER

The biggest mistake anyone could make would be to underestimate Thit. This quietly spoken, petite woman of Burmese background has a beautiful nature. When I heard her story and the way in which she has used her own cancer journey to help others, I was in awe of her accomplishments.

Thit had a long and stable 30 year career with the Department of Education. Starting as a High School Teacher, Thit moved on to write policy, then English as a Second Language (ESL) training, and then to administration as the Operations Manager for the NSW Adult Migrant English Service of two major regions in Sydney.

At age 62, Thit decided to retire as commuting everyday between Wollongong and Sydney was becoming too strenuous. It was time to enjoy retirement with her husband Kiet; and together, they travelled quite a bit over the following years. But this was not enough to keep Thit occupied. She wanted to do something significant that would make a difference in the world around her.

As a Burmese Muslim, Thit had noticed that since the 9/11 attacks in the US, there was a lot of unpleasantness among different religious groups and there seemed to be some inaccurate ideas about the Islamic faith. She aspired to open up a dialogue between religions and in 2010, with the help of local Council, Thit started the Illawarra Women's Interfaith Network (I-WIN). The purpose of I-WIN was to promote harmony, understanding and respect among followers of the various world religions.

The inaugural meeting was attended by women from the Bahá'i, Catholic, Interfaith, Islam, Buddhist, Jewish and Quaker faiths and, through a mixture of activities, the women were able break down prejudices and build bridges.

It was around this time that Thit's cancer journey began. A strong believer in early detection, she had had mammograms from the age of 50, never missing any of her biannual screenings. In all those years, her tests were clear, so when Thit went in for her scheduled appointment at age 66, she expected the same, and left for a trip overseas before getting the results. Upon her return, there was a message on her answering machine requesting her to go into the Breast Clinic.

It never crossed Thit's mind that there would be a problem. She self-examined her breasts regularly and there were no lumps. She was healthy; she did not drink, she did not smoke, and she had breastfed all three of her children. There was no reason to be worried, so she thought that the mammogram may have been done incorrectly.

Thit returned to the Breast Clinic the next morning where the staff informed her that they would need to do the mammogram again. Once the screening was complete, they asked her to stay.

"A psychologist came out and said to me, 'You know, we are looking at the mammogram. Don't get worked up because sometimes it's nothing and that's fine.' I wasn't worried at the time, not at all."

A little later, Thit was called into the doctor's office and told that she would need an ultrasound. That moment was accompanied by a memorable piece of inspiration.

"We were sitting there, and on the wall was this picture of a teacup. And on it was written: 'Women are like teabags,

they don't know how strong they are until they are in hot water.' I thought it was perfect! It was a brilliant thing. It is really true."

Following the ultrasound, Thit was advised that she should see the surgeon before she left. By this time, she had been at the clinic for four hours and she began to sense that something was wrong. Thit phoned Kiet and asked him to come in to support her. They were together when the surgeon conducted the examination and because he could not feel any lumps, the doctor asked her to stay for a biopsy.

"Up to that stage, I knew that there was something wrong, but there was always the high possibility that it might not be cancer. My mind was saying, 'I hope it's not cancer,' but after the biopsy was done, my morale was getting pretty low."

They returned to the surgeon a few days later for the results. Thit admits that she somehow knew, deep down inside, that it was not going to be good news. When she was diagnosed with invasive ductal carcinoma breast cancer, Thit became very silent. She was internalising the information and did not want to talk. Her mind was filled with all sorts of worries and imaginary outcomes and thoughts. It was Kiet who started shooting a lot of questions at the doctor. Being a university professor and researcher, Kiet immediately went online to research Thit's diagnosis and treatment. He said to her, "Everything will be fine, you do the operation and then it will be fine, no problems." Thit had seen several colleagues go through breast cancer and she knew it wasn't that simple.

"I couldn't get it into Kiet's head that this is not something that once you've done the operation, you'll be fine, or once you've done the treatment it will be fine...it is the rest of your life, it is a journey. I realised it then and there, I just felt it."

The reason that Thit and the doctors could not feel a lump was because it was right at the back on her chest wall. Without the mammogram and subsequent ultrasound, her tumour would never have been detected. The surgeon performed a lumpectomy and due to the location and spread of the cancer, Thit also had some lymph nodes removed, causing problems with her arm movement.

This was the first in a series of events that led Thit to do something to help other breast cancer patients. She was surprised that no one explained to her why she was having trouble with her arm, and further, what she could do to regain function. Thit had to discover for herself that physiotherapy was the solution and fortunately, after a few sessions, the movement in her arm was restored. She credits the Breast Cancer Network Australia (BCNA) Kit for providing this and other much needed information. Thit also began noticing a general attitude of prejudgement when people dealt with her.

"Even in the hospital, the doctor came up to me and asked the nurse, 'Does this lady speak English?' And I would say, 'Why don't you talk to her yourself?' It still happens. When I went to see another doctor, he took one look at me and asked, 'Do you need an interpreter?'"

The assumption that Thit was a non-English speaking migrant woman could not have been further from the truth. Her command of English is excellent, and her education and career credentials are second to none, yet the prejudice, intentional or not, still exists.

After surgery, her medical team recommended chemotherapy and radiation. Even though the 28 mm (1.1 in) tumour had been completely removed, the margins were small and the location, so deep in the chest, made it important to have these additional treatments.

For Thit, chemotherapy was horrific. She was administered her first dose of two drugs intravenously and went home, expecting to feel unwell for a few days, and then better from there. What actually happened was that on day four, Thit completely collapsed and her daughter Mimi, a radiation oncologist, took her to emergency where they discovered that Thit's whole immune system had shut down. She did not have any white blood cells in her body.

The medical staff gave her an injection to boost the production of white blood cells. She was admitted to an isolation ward and, almost immediately, a huge lump grew on the side of her neck, indicating an infection. Eventually it subsided and after a week, Thit recovered enough to go home, but her immune system was so compromised that shingles manifested and covered a quarter of her body.

The difficult question became how to administer the chemotherapy treatment. Thit was asked if she wanted to continue and she thought, "What a silly question, now that I've started." She said, "Yes, of course I will continue." To prevent another total system crash, her doctor reduced one drug by 10% and the other by 15% and arranged special permission for her to receive the expensive booster injection each time she had chemotherapy.

Thit was blessed to have family support in the form of her husband Kiet, her children Kim, Mimi and Tommy, and her sister Mila, who would come down from Sydney during her worst days of chemotherapy recovery. Because of the physical difficulty of her treatment, Thit realised that she needed to aid her recovery by focussing her mind on something other than herself.

There were two things that kept Thit positive. The first was finding a project, and she decided on creating a little Japanese garden. When she saw an ad for Zen Landscaping on the back of a supermarket docket, she took it as a sign and engaged the company to help her build it.

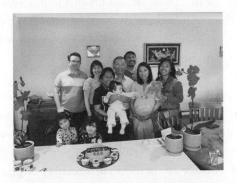

Thit with her family on her 70th birthday

"I had that project while I was going through chemo. I didn't have to do anything, I just sat there and said do this

and do that. It kept my focus away from myself. I was outdoors in the sunshine and when I was well enough, Kiet would drive me to different nurseries to purchase plants. That really helped to pull me through."

The second thing was her faith and spirituality.

"Because of my faith, Islam, we believe that when ailments happen, it is more or less like a cleansing of your sins. And if you have faith and you can count the blessings of what you have, that in itself is a way to cure you."

Thit feels strongly that her faith and positive attitude helped her to persevere throughout her health challenges. Instead of feeling sorry for herself, every day she would ask herself the question, "What is the blessing that I have today?" and she would write it in her diary like a gratitude journal. She wrote simple things, like, "The sun was so beautiful today," or, "My lovely friend phoned today." She chose to focus on the good, which she feels really helped her to heal.

Following chemotherapy, Thit had radiation therapy for a month. On one of her visits, she noticed that there was a meditation class being run by a psycho-oncologist. She thought it would be good to attend and learn something that could help her recovery. There were about 30 women in the class, and Thit immediately saw that she was the only non-white Australian person in the room. The facilitator began by suggesting that each of the attendees do some ice-breaking and talk to the person next to them.

"Everyone turned to someone else and I was just sitting there alone. That made me uncomfortable. The facilitator saw I was alone and came to speak to me. I asked, 'Where are the Asian and other nationalities who have cancer?' She said, 'Oh, they have their own community support.'"

That was not a good enough answer for Thit. As far as she knew, community cancer support groups for other cultures did not exist. She tried again to get support by attending a Breast Cancer Support Group and found that the same attitude prevailed. Normally, that sort of thing would not affect her but at the time, she felt vulnerable.

Thit felt the same judgement when she attended a Look Good, Feel Better workshop, an event designed to help cancer survivors with their skincare, make-up and wigs. Despite calling them prior to the event to inform them of her skin colouring, she felt annoyed at being ignored and angry about being treated like a second-class citizen.

These experiences ignited a spark in Thit that would become a bright, shining beacon for many women. She thought, "Wouldn't it be good to have a group that would be culturally sensitive so that people could feel safe and comfortable to come?"

Thit contacted her friend Vimala at the local Council who had assisted in setting up the interfaith network and talked to her about her experiences and the problems she had faced. She posed a number of questions to Vimala:

"Why are multi-cultural women's voices not being heard? Why aren't they using these services? The government provides so much money for all of that and if these women are not accessing them, it is such a waste of funding. Why are multicultural women so invisible in the cancer arena?"

Vimala asked Thit what she wanted to do, and at that stage, she had no idea, but she knew that she wanted to do something. Vimala suggested a meeting with representatives from the Cancer Council and the Multicultural Community Council of Illawarra (MCCI) and Area Health Services to discuss the issue.

These organisations came together and agreed to support Thit if she came up with a plan. Around the same time, the BCNA contacted her with an invitation to train as a Community Liaison Officer. She had just finished her radiation treatment, so she agreed to attend the three-day interstate event where she met women from all different backgrounds who had been through breast cancer journeys.

Thit's perspective grew from her personal view to the broader perspective of what other women experience and she returned home even more determined to do something.

A few days later, Thit was contacted by the president of the

Illawarra Muslim Women's Association to speak at their Big Morning Tea, a fundraising event held annually as an initiative by the Cancer Council. Thit knew many of the attendees because, prior to her cancer diagnosis, many of the women had attended her English classes.

Thit went along and shared her story to the group of Muslim women. She talked about her experiences and also asked the group why they were not accessing all the support programs currently offered by the government. Thit discovered that it was due to the same reasons behind her own feelings of discomfort. Some of the ladies asked if Thit would create something specifically for them.

"I am old and sick. I am 67 and not too well," said Thit. "There are a lot of things I can't do, and I would need young people to help me."

Right then and there, four young mothers came forward and offered to help. Thit took this as a sign, an answer to her prayers.

"Through my journey, I never asked, 'Why me?' I asked God, 'What are you trying to tell me? What is the message? What do you want me to do? I will do it.' That's what I kept on telling myself, 'I will do whatever needs to be done.'"

Thit's belief that everything happens for a reason propelled her to see a purpose. She was not a victim; her experience was a blessing that opened her eyes to a whole group of women she needed to help.

From that simple beginning came the Sisters' Cancer Support Group (SCSG). With the help of the Council in providing a hall; the BCNA assisting with marketing; and the generosity of the community in the form of suppliers including Print Media and a photographer, the SCSG launched in 2014 with more than 70 people in attendance.

The SCSG supports women from Multicultural and Muslim backgrounds who have cancer or supporting a loved one who has cancer. The group draws on a holistic care model to provide social, emotional and spiritual support to promote healing and wellness.

When the group started, the challenge Thit faced was to break through the silence. Within the Muslim, Turkish, Lebanese and Arabic communities, there is a very strong stigma attached to talking about cancer. At the first meeting, there were some women who were very upset because they had experienced cancer or had lost someone to cancer, but they just felt that they could not speak. Thit had to work out a way to open up communication and she began by holding an information session.

The SCSG team organised childcare, food and a Turkish and Arabic translator. Thit shared her personal story and used pictures to convey emotions to work around any language barriers. Once the women felt safe, they began to share and the SCSG has met every month since its launch and continues to do so. Today the meetings are held at the MCCI and they are open to all. Thit has ladies from Libya, Syria, Lebanon, Morocco and Africa in attendance. The majority of these women wear headscarves and would not have felt comfortable to go anywhere else for support.

In 2017, the SCSG became a registered organisation and it is the first multicultural-specific support group in Australia. It received the Community Innovation award from the MCCI for services provided to the community.

Thit used her extensive management skills to ensure that the organisation was set up properly and with the full support of medical professionals. The SCSG has an advisory committee of highly respected individuals and enjoys the backing of the Cancer Council, the BCNA, the Multicultural Health Service, Wollongong City Council and the MCCI.

In the same year, the SCSG also received funding from the Cancer Institute for Project SAHA (Survivorship, Awareness, Healthy Living, Access), a video series focussed on how cancer survivors are successfully living well after treatment. This is becoming an increasingly important issue as more and more people are surviving after cancer. Knowing what to do during treatment is as simple as following the doctor's instructions, but after it is finished, keeping healthy to ensure that cancer does not return can be the most challenging part.

There is no doubt that the SCSG will continue to thrive. Thit feels that she has been led to do this work, to teach women, many of whom do not speak English, how to eat and live well after cancer. Her contribution to the cancer community was honoured with an invitation to be an ambassador for the Cancer Council Relay for Life.

Thit's work with the SCSG has been so successful that she has been asked to replicate her efforts in the Sydney region. She continues to inspire and bless women on their cancer journey, a true example of how cancer saves lives.

"To live you need to have a will to live and secondly, you need to have purpose. My purpose has been with my children. Before it was work and family, and when work finished, it was just the family, and now it is my family and my Sisters' Cancer Support Group. I am grateful that I am making a difference."

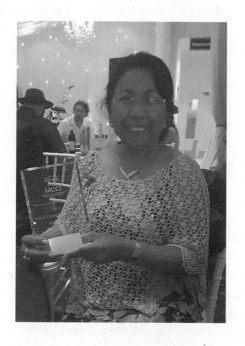

10

LISA, AARON, JOSH, BEN, ELLA, ROSE, MYLES

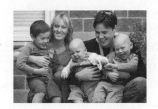

DIAGNOSIS: NEPHROBLASTOMA WILMS' TUMOUR

Aaron and Lisa's happy and busy life with their children is both joyful and inspiring when you know the story of their family's cancer journey.

I felt an instant connection with Lisa when I met her: she is a striking, confident woman who has accomplished the admirable feat of combining a long and successful corporate career with a wonderful personal life. Lisa worked her way up the corporate ladder in the field of Human Resources within the Technology sector, during her twenties. Single and with her thirtieth birthday looming, Lisa felt that she might be "left on the shelf." As it turned out, she soon met the love of her life, Aaron and they knew they were meant to find each other.

Even though he has lived in Australia for 20 years, Aaron retains his Kiwi accent and staunch support for the All Blacks. Of Maori descent, family has always been an important part of his life. He is a great father, as evidenced by the close relationship he has with his children.

Aaron had a successful career in logistics management. He had always wanted a big family, a desire that Lisa shared. Told by many that falling pregnant can take time, they started 'practising' before their

March 2001 wedding and Lisa walked down the aisle 19 weeks pregnant.

The gorgeous, healthy Josh was born "just this perfect child." Lisa took a short maternity leave and had to go back to work as they needed two incomes to pay their mortgage. One night when Josh was a few months old, Lisa was home breastfeeding him when she had a sudden urge for a Big Mac, Large Fries, Apple Pie and a Chocolate Sundae. Aaron was dumbfounded as Lisa never eats McDonalds.

Eight months after that craving, the super fertile Lisa gave birth naturally to Benjamin, a big baby boy weighing in at 5.83 kg (12 lb 10 oz). Josh had also been a big baby at 4.62 kg (10 lb 4 oz). The petite Sri Lankan obstetrician who delivered Ben nearly dropped him because he was so huge! The midwives were so surprised and excited to borrow Ben for "show and tell" with the growing audience that had heard about this super-sized baby in the birthing ward.

Ben was born 64 cm (25.2 in) long, way above the average length, and he was black and blue because he had been crammed inside Lisa's uterus. At the time, they attributed his size, weight and colour to Aaron's Maori heritage, but they discovered later that it was because of an 'overgrowth' gene and part of a hereditary genetic cancer.

Lisa and Aaron were excited to have their family growing but when Ben was around 18 months, they noticed that he had a distended tummy. As Lisa cuddled him one night, she felt a hard lump the size of a tennis ball in his stomach.

First thing the next morning, Lisa and her mother took Ben straight to the hospital where they performed an ultrasound. Within a few minutes, they were told that there appeared to be a tumour and they were referred to an oncologist at Westmead Children's Hospital.

Later that same day, little Ben was diagnosed with Stage 4 nephroblastoma or Wilms' tumour, a cancer of the kidneys that typically occurs in children. Lisa and Aaron were devastated.

"At the start, the doctor said it could go on for three or four years. I remember thinking, 'That's like climbing Mount Everest. We're never going to get there.' But then, when I look back at it now, we made it. We made it through."

— AARON

Ben's oncologist was a source of sound medical and practical advice. Having worked with many families of sick children, he advised against making any drastic life changes and to focus on establishing a plan of action.

Ben was admitted to hospital the same day he was diagnosed. With Josh to take care of as well as their responsibilities to their respective jobs, Aaron kept working and taking care of Josh. He came back and forth to the hospital while Lisa stayed in the ward with Ben.

The couple embarked on a steep learning curve to become educated on Wilms' tumour and the prescribed treatment. This knowledge was essential for them figure out how to fit their lives around the surgery and all the regular hospital visits that would be required. Lisa felt totally exhausted.

"I thought it was the heavy weight of the news on me, the emotional drain. I was so tired I could barely move."

— LISA

On Ben's second day in hospital, Lisa woke up and called Aaron, asking him to arrange for her Mum to look after Josh so he could come to the hospital. They talked to the doctors, discussed the procedure and then, as they were both so emotionally and physically spent, they both fell asleep with Ben in his hospital room.

Lisa woke first, with an odd feeling. For some reason she was compelled to go downstairs to the hospital pharmacy and purchase a pregnancy test. She went into the bathroom, did the test and emerged just as Aaron was stirring, and announced, "I've got some news for you. We're pregnant."

A rollercoaster of emotions flooded through both of them. How could all of this happen in the space of two days? It was overwhelming, just too much to process. They were thrilled to be having another child, but because of Ben's diagnosis, their immediate thought was, "What if this is genetic?"

Wilms' tumour is a hereditary and genetic cancer. As a toddler, Aaron had the same disease and even though they had mentioned it when asked about familial illnesses in the early stages of pregnancy, they were told that it was unlikely to be hereditary.

"Shame they said that. If they had told us there was even just the tiniest percentage chance that it was hereditary, we would have checked. Hindsight can be cruel."

— LISA

Aaron had been only two years old when he was taken to hospital and diagnosed with Wilms' tumour. The medical team at Auckland Hospital removed one kidney and he also had chemotherapy. Being so young, the memory that stood out the most for Aaron was standing up in the hospital crib and howling as his parents left him there. Back in the 1970s, parents did not stay in hospital with their children whereas today, parents are welcomed and supported.

"I remember feeling a lot of guilt because I had had it. I knew that it was too much of a coincidence for it to be just random bad luck. But we had to put our feelings aside so that we could make the right decisions for Ben. You can't do that if you are walking around thinking, 'Why has the world done this to us?' You have to get past that and be positive and think about what is required."

— AARON

When Ben was diagnosed, it was the early 2000's, back when the internet and Google was in its infancy. Fast forward 15 years to the access we now have to an infinite amount of information, and who knows, Lisa and Aaron may have been able to research Ben's condition for themselves before he was born—a re-examination of Ben's ultrasound in utero showed that he had kidneys the size of a 10-year-old child.

Ben had surgery immediately, removing almost all of one kidney and most of the other. This was followed by chemotherapy, including trials of new drugs that had just become available. He also had radiation and they thought he was doing well, when more tumours appeared, and he had to undergo further surgery.

"He was only a bubba, 18 months, and he was very brave."

— Lisa

Ben was fitted with a central line to administer the chemotherapy, and sometimes he got an infection. With his immune system so compromised, any bacteria in the air could cause an infection and result in hospitalisation. He was in and out of hospital constantly and this was unsettling for the whole family. Aaron told me about one particular day when he took Ben in for a routine blood test.

"He loved to ride on my shoulders. After the test, we hadn't walked 20 metres and he must have picked up a bug in his lines, because he was all happy when I put him up there and then I just noticed his head falling down past my head, it was that quick. I had another 75 metres to the oncology ward, and by the time I got there, he was in my arms. We didn't leave the hospital for two weeks and I called Lisa to bring us some clothes."

— Aaron

To make things easier, they sometimes lived at Westmead Hospital for periods of time and got to know other families with sick children. Lisa remarked on the number of parents there alone with no support and the many single parents whose marriages had crumbled under the strain of caring for a very ill child. Her heart went out to these parents, coping with the overwhelming emotional strain while having to deal with the practical financial and day-to-day functions of caring for their healthy children.

"You've got to remain strong for all the children, for each other. I couldn't completely lose it and then leave it to

Aaron. He wouldn't do that to me either. And as much as we had sick children, we wanted to have happy children."

— Lisa

During pregnancy with Ella, the doctors would not diagnose her in utero, but they did keep measuring her kidneys. This caused Lisa and Aaron to strongly suspect that Ella had the same gene.

Ella was born early at 37 weeks, 5.11 kg (11 lb 10 oz). With a smile, Lisa recounted to me her experience in the premature ward where all the other parents had these tiny 20 cm (7.8 in) babies while Ella was too long for the humidicrib—they had to take the top off "like a fish tank" so she could fit into it. She felt the questioning stares and knew they were wondering what she was doing in there with a baby that was 10 times the size of theirs! Lisa and Aaron came to understand that this 'overgrowth' syndrome was symptomatic of Wilms' tumour. Aaron and Ella both still show the effects of that genetic product.

Once Ella was born, they could see tumours growing, and diagnosed her with the same cancer. Ella had her first and only operation to remove pieces of her kidney at three months of age. She then began a chemotherapy regime that continued right up until she was four years old. It was a real challenge to coordinate Ben and Ella's treatments and look after Josh. Aaron and Lisa knew that something needed to change. Aaron explained their thoughts at the time:

"We needed to make things better for the family, for the kids. We had two kids needing treatment. One would be in hospital, then you would get out of there and the other one would be in. It was too tough, so we made the decision for me to stop working. It was family first and it was definitely the right thing to do."

— Aaron

Keeping positive during that time was a conscious decision that Lisa and Aaron chose to make every day.

"We wanted to make sure that every day they got up, our children were enjoying life. We didn't know how long their lives were going to be, we didn't know if Ella was going to make it, we thought that we were going to be able to save Ben and we couldn't. It was all unknown. What we did know was that we could get up every day and make their life as happy as possible."

— LISA

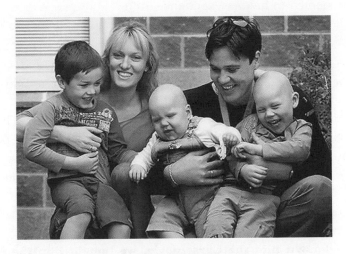

Lisa and Aaron with Josh, Ella and Ben

The family was blessed to have a supportive group of friends who were very generous. Within days of Ben's diagnosis and right through the following years, meals turned up to fill their freezer. Much appreciated help was provided with babysitting and transport, even though many of these friends were themselves couples with young children.

When Ben was four years old, Lisa was away on an overseas work trip. Just before boarding a plane for home, she called Aaron, who told her that Ben had been sitting on the lounge for a few days and he was not himself. Aaron felt that they needed to take him to hospital and Lisa agreed.

Arriving home 24 hours later, Lisa saw that Ben was very deflated and tired. It was the 19th of December when they took him into hospital for two days of tests. Eventually, the doctors reached the point where they told Lisa and Aaron that there was nothing else they could do. They said that the important thing was to make him comfortable until he passed away. It was hard news to take.

> **"Even though we knew he had gotten worse, we always lived in hope that something would happen, that somehow he would pull through."**
>
> — Lisa

Lisa and Aaron immediately looked at each other and said that they wanted to take him home. The doctor advised them to bring the family's Christmas celebration forward, which they did.

Christmas was held on the 22nd of December that year. They had all the trimmings: a wonderful meal, exchanging and opening presents and, most importantly, Ben had all of his family around him.

The hospital provided a plan to manage Ben's pain, with morphine, oxygen and a palliative care nurse. He was not eating, and he did not want to sleep. He just wanted to watch Sailor Moon DVDs.

> **"We bought him the Cars movie, we bought him the car from the movie actually, hoping that he might get some energy in his last few days, but he didn't. He was ready to go."**
>
> — Lisa

Ben didn't get off the lounge in those last few days. Lisa sat with him, reading books and massaging him because she was worried that he was going to be sore and uncomfortable from not moving. It finally got to the stage where Ben was getting very sick, finding it difficult to breathe because the tumours that had spread to his lungs were growing larger and the growth could not be stopped.

Aaron and Lisa were prepared for this stage. They agreed with the palliative care nurse that now was the time to administer oxygen, so they talked to Ben about what they needed to do. The nurse came over and Ben just said, "I don't want it."

> **"He made the decision he wanted to go. We had to respect that, so we actually didn't give him any oxygen. He wanted to go, so we got the whole family to come and, one by one, talk to him and say their goodbyes. We had our grandparents, aunties, uncles, you name it, we had a houseful of people. And the kids, and Josh, poor Josh, I don't think he really knew what was going on. Ella was 18 months and she had no idea what was going on."**
>
> — LISA

Lisa recalled the incredibly touching moment when Ella, who was just learning to talk, said Ben's name for the first time when it was her turn to say goodbye. It is a memory that Lisa and Aaron will always treasure.

They held Ben and stayed with him until he passed away.

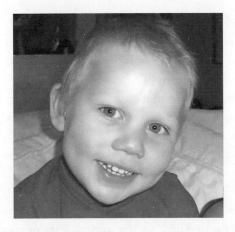

Ben

Aaron and Lisa were very aligned in the way they dealt with Ben's passing. They were grateful that they were able to spend time with him, to say goodbye and respect his wishes, but because they also had Josh and Ella to consider, they made a conscious decision to create a happy family and not to drown in sadness.

The hospital offered counselling support, but neither of them were ready for it.

"A child dying at that age, they're just a baby. They have their whole life ahead of them. He was such a brave little boy who died so young. For me, that's just the worst thing that could have ever happened. For me, you couldn't throw anything more awful at me now in life because the worst thing that could ever happen to a mother has happened to me. To be honest, it's taken away my fear of dying. I felt numb when he passed away. I felt numb for many, many years and whilst it was never diagnosed, when I spoke to a counsellor later on, he did say to me that I was most likely going through post-traumatic stress. I am still processing and grieving."

— LISA

Looking back, Lisa concedes that it might have been beneficial to have had some counselling, but they were only just keeping their heads above water and trying to manage and balance work, paying the bills, and keeping their kids happy. The couple just did not have time to stop and grieve. Between work, making time for the kids, and going back and forth to the hospital with Ella, it was a logistical nightmare, but they got through it.

Aaron feels that his grieving process started when Ben was first diagnosed.

"When Ben did pass away, the family was already somewhat conditioned to the news. I'm not saying it was easy, or anything like that. I'm grateful for the time we got

**to spend with him. If you are going to lose a kid, this was
better than losing him all of a sudden."**

— AARON

Part of Aaron's coping strategy was writing a regular email
newsletter for friends and family. When he started, he sent it out to 12
people, but the distribution list kept growing and by the end it was up
to around 60!

Aaron found that writing down his thoughts was therapeutic. Aaron
and Lisa believe that sharing their story, being open and transparent,
answering questions honestly, and talking about Ben has been their way
of dealing with their grief.

One of the hardest things was going back to the hospital for Ella's
treatment, without Ben.

**"Normally, when parents are going through that, they have
one child and it either turns out well, or it turns out badly.
When things go well, they have good memories. If things
turn out badly, you don't have to go back. Things turned out
badly for us, but we had to take Ella back for treatment the
week after Ben's funeral and for years after that."**

— AARON

Every time they walked through the doors at The Children's
Hospital, a flood of sad memories washed over them. Fifteen years on,
it still hits them. Aaron had formed friendships with many of the other
parents and noticed that they treated him differently after Ben passed.

**"People asked where Ben was, and we had to tell them. I
could sense that they stopped coming up and talking to me
like they normally would because I became a reminder of
the negative side and of course they wanted to keep their
kid in a positive environment."**

— AARON

Even the medical team had difficulty in dealing with the family because every time they came in for treatment with Ella, they were reminded of Ben, one of the few children they had lost to Wilms' tumour.

Ella is now 12 years old and has not needed to have any further treatment since she finished chemotherapy at age four. There are no signs of any side-effects from her treatment, however she is regularly checked and closely monitored.

Lisa and Aaron credit Ben for saving Ella's life. If they had not gone through the journey with Ben, they might have lost Ella. Because Ben was diagnosed when they were pregnant with Ella, it saved her life.

Despite their emotional journey, Lisa and Aaron maintained their ideal of a large and happy family. The genetics team at Westmead Hospital took an interest in their case and asked them to become the subject of a project on familial cancer. The team partnered with the Royal Melbourne Institute of Technology (RMIT University) to study their family history and genetics to discover how the gene was passed on.

Blood samples were taken from every member of their family, as well as extended family both in Australia and New Zealand. The study was able to detect the gene that caused the cancer and they discovered that it did not come from the Maori side of the family as they had originally thought. The gene actually came through Aaron's grandmother's line of Anglo-Saxon heritage. She was a blue-eyes blonde with fair skin and married Aaron's grandfather who is of Maori heritage. Their son, Aaron's Dad, also married a blue-eyed blonde, and then Aaron married Lisa, yet another blue-eyed blonde. The men in Aaron's family definitely have a type!

Once the team isolated the gene, they offered Lisa and Aaron the opportunity to conceive via In Vitro Fertilisation (IVF), working in partnership with Sydney IVF in order to screen out the embryos with the gene before implanting them. In their first round, they created eight embryos and five of them had the cancer gene. From the three healthy embryos, Lisa and Aaron welcomed Rose into the world.

"Rose was our gift, she was our little miracle. You're so sad

when you lose a child. It was a gift that we were able to have more."

— LISA

When Lisa turned 40, the couple decided to try once more and they created six embryos, three with the cancer gene, and three healthy. One of those healthy embryos became their son Myles Benjamin.

There was a lot of pressure during Lisa's pregnancy with Myles. I could tell I was about to hear a funny story as Lisa's serious words were accompanied with a smile.

"Josh came up to Aaron and me. He was about seven, maybe eight. He walked right up and said, 'You know, Mum and Dad, I really want a baby brother.' How's that for pressure? Because he'd lost Ben, he now just had two sisters and really wanted a brother."

— LISA

Josh is now 16, and Myles is eight. Josh dotes on his new little buddy. He is his rugby coach and his baseball coach—Myles idolises his big brother Josh.

As we sat around their kitchen bench and chatted with the kids coming in and out of the room, my admiration for Aaron and Lisa grew immeasurably. This family has come through the worst possible trauma and emerged as a strong, loving, thriving unit.

"We always say there is a missing piece of our family. We're always talking about Ben, even Rose and Myles talk about him all the time and ask a lot of questions. We have pictures around the house and he's still very much a part of the family."

— LISA

"I'm not going to say it was hard. It was just something we had to do. If you are in our situation, remain positive. Listen to your doctors. Continue to enjoy your child. Try not to make it a focal point of your life and keep doing the fun things that kids want to do. It's too easy to get overwhelmed with the darkness and gravity of the situation. Spend time with your kids and try to give them a normal life."

— AARON

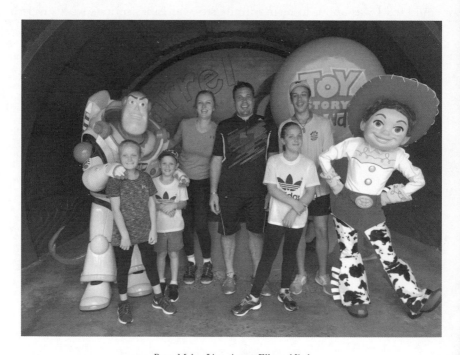

Rose, Myles, Lisa, Aaron, Ella and Josh

"You can't just fall into a hole. I have to pull myself up consciously all the time and tell myself to live life today. When you go through these things, it builds your resilience and it changes how you respond to the world and approach life."

— LISA

11

JOHN

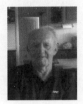

DIAGNOSIS: LUNG AND ADRENAL CANCER

John and his wife Margaret are a laconic, 'salt of the earth' couple who have been married for 55 years. Their love for each other has only strengthened through life's challenges. Witnessing their deep love and care for one another was truly inspiring.

The two met and married when they were teenagers. Margaret gave birth to Teresa at age 16; to Katie one year later; and to Jason at age 21. The young couple struggled when Katie was diagnosed with Muscular Dystrophy and they nursed her until she passed aged 13. John worked extra shifts at the brickworks and started working a second job to support the family. He began employment at the spinning mill where he continued to work for many years until he retired decades later as under manager.

John is now 76 years old. Until four years ago, he was healthy and well, so when he started coughing up blood, he simply ignored it. There was a lot going on at the time—Margaret's mother, who was suffering from Parkinson's disease, had been admitted to hospital after a long battle with the illness, and her prognosis did not look good.

John was loath to bother Margaret about a little blood, so he did not say anything for about a month. It took a persistent sore on his forehead to finally motivate him to see a doctor.

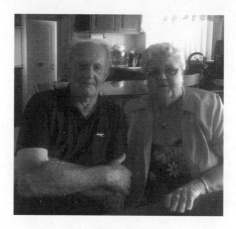

John and Margaret

John's GP checked his head and gave him something to heal the sore. As an afterthought, John mentioned that he had been coughing up blood. His doctor immediately sent him off for a CT scan.

A few days later, John was called back for the results, and the couple went to the appointment on their way to see Margaret's mother. John was told that he had an aggressive cancer in the bottom of his left lung. I asked him how he felt when he found out the news.

"Well, I didn't feel on top of the world. This might sound strange, but I thought, 'This is not going to happen to me.' I used to smoke, but I gave it up more than 20 years ago. I didn't feel good about it, but I was more worried about Margaret."

Margaret's eyes teared up as John's words took her back to that time.

"We went to visit Margaret's mother straight after and she died that night. So, Margaret had a double whammy, she had me diagnosed with cancer that day, and her mother died that night."

Margaret was in tears for days, it was just too much for her to process. They had nursed Margaret's mother for six years and it was traumatic to see her body give out while her mind was still sharp.

It was up to Margaret to make funeral arrangements and sort out her mother's affairs. She described how difficult that was with John's diagnosis looming over them:

"Between diagnosis and John's operation, it was about three months. We had to arrange Mum's funeral, clean out her flat and do all that before he could go to hospital because I had no other family to help me. It was so hard because John was so sick, and I was watching him like a hawk."

At diagnosis, John's tumour was the size of a golf ball. By the time of the operation, it had grown aggressively to the size of a tennis ball. He was lucky that the tumour was located in an isolated position because if it had been in the top half of his lungs near the airways, it could have spread all over his body.

The other piece of luck was that his PET scan showed that the rest of his body appeared to be cancer-free. Due to John's age, if there had been another cancer site, he thinks that his prognosis would have been entirely different.

John was given some basic information on his forthcoming operation.

"I looked at it and the first thing it said was that only 15% of the people who have this operation live for five years. I said, 'That's it. I'm not going to read this. I don't want to know any more,' and I didn't read any further."

John trusted his medical team and was admitted to hospital for the operation. His surgeon performed a thoracotomy to access his lungs. This was combined with a lobectomy to remove the tumour.

Margaret was waiting for him in ICU after the surgery and she described the drama that ensued.

"I nearly lost him three times that first night. He came out of surgery and he was breathing by a machine, he had tubes coming out everywhere. He got a staphylococcus infection and three mornings out of the 10, I walked in and they pulled me up and told me that they nearly lost him through the night. The last time they said that the doctor and two nurses had fought all night to keep him alive."

Despite these close calls, John pulled through and after 10 days he was released from ICU into a regular ward. I asked him if he remembered how he felt during that critical time when his life was hanging in the balance.

"When I was lying there with all the gear hanging out of me, I didn't tell Margaret, but I thought to myself, 'If I just live for another three years, I'll be fine.' I love fishing and I just wanted to get down and do a bit more fishing."

Like many of the other survivors in this book, John found his reason to live. In that moment, it was fishing that motivated him to fight for his life.

After a couple of days in a regular ward, the doctor discharged John from hospital into Margaret's care.

"They went in through my back, through my ribs. They had to break ribs and take all the nerves, so I had bad pain for a couple of years. It's gone now, but if I touch the area, there's just a numb feeling."

Once his wounds were healed, John went back for his check-up and found that his doctors had contradictory views on his follow-up treatment. The surgeon had suggested he would not need chemotherapy. When he saw his own doctor, he suggested going to the cancer clinic to have radiotherapy.

When John arrived to have radiation, the oncologist recommended chemotherapy, citing the evidence that people who underwent chemotherapy after John's type of operation tended to live longer. The doctor assured him that there was no cancer present but recommended that he should still undergo chemotherapy as a preventative measure.

John and Margaret respected the doctor's advice and decided to go ahead with chemotherapy. Unfortunately, the treatment caused some serious side-effects.

His regime was set at once a week for three months. After the first dose, John got so sick that, 24 hours later, Margaret had to call an ambulance to take him to hospital.

The most unusual side-effect was a terrible clanging sound inside John's head, like two pieces of metal banging together over and over again. Margaret verified that she could hear it when she put her ear near his head and so did his doctor. What was making the sound and how it was possible remains a mystery. John's doctor changed his chemotherapy drug and the clanging did stop, but his other symptoms continued.

"I was still in bad pain and after every dose, I would physically collapse and end up back in hospital for four or five days until my white cell count came back up."

This stretched his treatment regime out to fortnightly for six months. John remembers spending that time on the lounge at home, pasty white and painfully thin.

"People would come and visit me, and I was just too crook, too sick to talk. I didn't want any visitors."

Margaret was very protective of John, and before anyone entered their home, she would check to see if the visitor had a cold or any other sickness. If a visitor was ill, she would ask them to come back when they were healthy. There was no way she was going to risk John catching another infection.

After the chemotherapy, John did recover, but the one side-effect that remained was his loss of all the nerves in his feet. This is something that he has come to terms with, even though it affects his favourite pastime.

"I would still have done chemo knowing the consequences to my feet. I can walk fine on flat ground, but I was a mad fisherman and I can't do that anymore."

John continued with his three-monthly check-ups and when his scans were all clear, they were increased to six-monthly intervals.

Everything was going well until Christmas 2016. A new scan revealed that the same aggressive cancer had returned, but it was showing in his adrenal gland. John's medical team informed him that he was a very unusual situation. Cancers like the one John had usually return as metastatic cancer, but John's reoccurrence was instead isolated in the one organ.

This was good news because it meant that the surgeon could eradicate the cancer by removing John's whole adrenal gland. He was admitted swiftly to ensure the operation occurred before the cancer spread any further. John was thankful that the procedure was performed with keyhole surgery, a minimally invasive operation compared to his first experience.

John has fully recovered and speaks philosophically about the remaining effects of his treatment:

"As far as the nerves in my feet go, there are people who have their whole life in a wheelchair and they still have a life. It might not be the same as someone who can run the 100-metre dash, but it's still a life."

John may not be able to climb rocks and fish on boats anymore, but he is grateful to be able to walk and drive unaided.

As he looks toward the future, John is not worried for himself. Margaret, his greatest supporter, is his main concern. Margaret does not drive, so he is thinking about selling the home they love to move closer to transport. He cites the assistance of friends and family in shuttling Margaret back and forth to the hospital as "one of the small things that was the biggest help."

I asked John for some advice for people facing their own cancer journey. This prompted a hilarious true story from his childhood that holds much wisdom.

When John was a child, he used to play on the vacant lots near his home. At age eight, he was running through the bush and trod on a tiger snake. It was dead and so rotten that he skidded. John raced home and yelled, "Dad! I'm poisoned! I can feel it coming up my leg!" He was utterly stressed out and convinced that he was going to die. John's Dad said, "Snake fright is worse than snake bite." He explained that sometimes when people get bitten by a snake, even a non-venomous snake, they can have a heart attack and die from the fright of the experience rather than the actual snake bite.

"A lot of people get sicker from worrying about it than from the actual cancer. Just take it easy. Go with how your body feels and do what you want to do. If you have to have chemo, have it, but it's up to you."

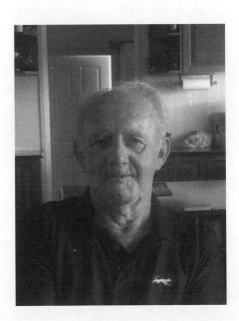

12

NINA

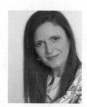

DIAGNOSIS: BREAST CANCER

Nina is a dynamic woman with a genuine heart for helping others. She is a brilliant fundraiser and, as Regional Development Manager NSW/ACT for the Leukaemia Foundation, she managed and directed exceptionally successfully fundraising campaigns.

Her entire career has been focussed on service and for the last 20 years, Nina has had a major impact in the field of health care, making a difference to many people's lives. Her accomplishments are due to her professionalism and hard work, but also to her beautiful spirit. Every time I see her, I feel Nina's heartfelt connection and it is this that sets her apart.

Being involved in the world of cancer, Nina is well-versed in the treatment and journeys of cancer patients. Her first encounter with the disease was when her grandmother passed from breast cancer at the age of 51. Back then, detection was poor, treatment options were limited and Nina wonders if many cases went undiagnosed.

Nina's own personal story is a wonderful example of being a cancer thriver. Her honesty and candour provide a real insight into how cancer affects our lives.

In 2005, about a year after the birth of her daughter, Nina noticed some lumps in her breast. She was not unduly concerned, thinking that she was young and that it was simply a hormonal response. However, she did have it checked by a specialist whose diagnosis was inflamed glands. He assured her that everything was fine and prescribed a six-month course of anti-inflammatory medication.

Fast forward five years later to Easter 2010 when her family was preparing to go on a camping trip. As she was getting undressed, she discovered some lumps, but they felt different than before and when she pressed on them, they just did not feel right.

Nina was happy to avoid the camping trip for an appointment with her GP, and upon examining the lumps, her doctor expressed concern and referred Nina to the same specialist she had visited five years prior about the same condition. This was followed by a series of tests: a CT scan, mammogram, ultrasound and a fine needle biopsy which all took place just before the Easter public holidays.

"I lived that whole weekend not knowing what was going on. I lived through every possible emotion, thinking, 'I've got cancer' to, 'Of course it's not.' I was numb, and I didn't want to talk about it, I didn't want to think about it."

The following Tuesday, Nina received a telephone call. She remembers being in the bathroom and hearing over the phone, "Mrs Field, don't panic but I'm sorry to say that your test results are back, and you have cancer." Nina's immediate thought was, "I knew that," but of course there was still a part of her that was hopeful.

"I wasn't shocked. It was more a case of how bad and what do I have to do. Am I going to die tomorrow, or what?"

Nina was diagnosed with a low-grade breast cancer but because the lumps had been growing for over five years, they had multiplied. Nina tells me that because she was 35 years old at the time, the density of her breast tissue meant that the mammogram did not pick up the cancerous lumps. Even the fine needle biopsy did not show that two of the lumps were cancerous.

"The key thing for me in all of this is that you have to listen to your body. Most of the time, there will be some kind of indication when you just know something is not right. I know you can't feel cancer, but I felt something was not right."

Her specialist asked if she wanted the facts, or if she needed it sugar-coated. Nina is naturally an emotional soul, but she also likes her information black and white. The doctor gave her the statistics and the probability of success for each option which allowed her to make an informed decision.

Nina was swiftly booked into surgery for a lumpectomy of the one lump that was positively identified as cancerous. On the morning of her surgery, she felt uneasy about the other two lumps and in the interim since consulting with the surgeon, she had decided that she wanted all three lumps removed, regardless of what the fine needle biopsy had revealed.

"I asked him to hook the other two out while he was in there. They were already cutting me open, so I wanted him to take it all. It became a drama to get clearance from the specialist, but they did it. It was only when those lumps were excised and tested that it was discovered that they were all cancerous, which meant I had to go back again and have another surgery to cut larger margins. It was awful because it could have been avoided."

In hindsight, Nina wonders if a mastectomy may have been a better option. She finds it difficult to find bras that fit and do not cause pain as she developed nerve damage from the multiple surgeries.

After her wounds had healed, Nina was required to undergo both chemotherapy and radiation. Her chemotherapy was scheduled at three weekly cycles and there were complications with Nina being neutropenic. Nina arranged to have chemotherapy in her own home as an outpatient. This proved to be a good decision due to the side-effects she suffered, including extreme tiredness and dreadful bone pain, "inside her bones."

"I remember I was just so tired and everything hurt. I had slow release pain patches, I lost so much weight, and at one stage I was so exhausted it was hard to breathe."

Nina's parents were incredibly supportive and helpful in caring for her children Josh and Maya, aged seven and six respectively at the time. During each cycle of chemotherapy, Nina's parents would take the children home with them on her worst days. Nina recalls a real turning point when she was struggling to breathe, and her kind, gentle father was worried and wanted to take her to hospital. She asked him to just open the window and to leave because it was so hard to watch his pain as a parent.

"I just wanted him to leave me alone at that moment. Sometimes we need to feel rubbish by ourselves."

Despite her physical pain, Nina found that one of the most mentally draining parts of her journey was having to keep reassuring everyone around her that she was okay. Well-meaning friends and family would say things like, "It will be okay," "You're okay." Whilst she loved them dearly, in her mind she was thinking, "Really? I am so not."

Nina finally snapped and said to one person, "I know you love me but stop saying that because I know you want me to be okay, but things are not okay."

Communicating honestly with friends and family is something Nina believes is vital for anyone undergoing cancer treatment. Her candid advice to be frank and open about how you feel and what you need is so essential. It enables your support team to understand how they can best help you.

"It's really important to have that open communication with friends to say, 'You know what, you can't fix me, I don't feel good, I'm hurting like hell. I'm okay with you not knowing what to do but don't tippy toe around me, just treat me like you normally would. Take me for a drive, because I can't drive. I'm starving but everything tastes awful except chips, so sit, eat chips and watch trash

TV with me because I can't concentrate to do anything else!'"

Nina, as with many other cancer survivors, found that in her time of crisis, those she thought would be pillars of strength were not there for her, and yet unexpected kindness came from many other people.

"Cancer is a very kind world, people are so kind when you have cancer."

It was the practical day-to-day tasks that Nina appreciated the most: meals for her family, picking up her children and sometimes entertaining and looking after them. This was especially valuable as, even before cancer, Nina and her husband knew their marriage was not working. They had tried to mend it, but it was not to be. Nina feels that she went through her cancer journey by herself.

"I guess it is hard to care for someone when you don't love them. When I got sick, there was almost another part of me grieving because I knew this was it. This is not going to work because we're here now, so some days I didn't know which was harder: my marriage ending or the cancer."

Nina recovered from chemotherapy and was excited to resume the school run, making a big effort to look well. She had always been a bit of a fashionista and loved to cover her bald head with pretty scarves. She recalls walking into the school yard and feeling the good wishes of all the Mums who would say, "You look so well," to which she would reply, "Yes, it's the cancer glow." It was her way to joke, keeping things light and normal for her children.

Nina is an amazing mother and she wanted to minimise the impact of her illness. She had changed from being a super active Mum to a Mum who not only looked different but felt different physically and emotionally. Josh and Maya are beautiful children; Nina's eyes twinkle as she lovingly shares how they would say, "Mum, you look so good," even when her head was bald, and she felt awful.

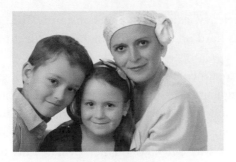

Josh, Maya and Nina

Radiation became the next challenge. Nina faced six weeks of radiation and after week four, she started to get burns. For Nina, that was not the worst part because she has a strong aversion to tattoos. It is standard practice for medical staff to tattoo marks on patients so that they can line up the body for radiation. She shows me the blue dots that are a permanent reminder of her treatment.

"I'm so anti-tattoos and every time I look in the mirror I see it. It was only a small dot, but I was so upset about it. Give me chemo but don't put on a tattoo. People have issues with hair loss, I didn't. I just didn't want the tattoo."

Following radiation therapy, Nina was prescribed Tamoxifen, however she could not tolerate the side-effects and eventually switched to slow-release pellets injected into her stomach for two years.

Nina also experienced the common but rarely discussed chemotherapy side-effect of 'chemo brain.' As a bright and intelligent woman, slowed brain function, the inability to access memory instantly and difficulty engaging motor skills for driving was distressing.

"It's like a fog you are reaching into. It's so frustrating, and then the frustration adds to it, it's like a vicious circle. My cognitive function was severely affected, and I had chemo brain, loss of memory during treatment."

For Nina, post-cancer treatment resulted in many other changes in her body: early menopause, hemochromatosis, fibromyalgia and a

Vitamin D deficiency, causing her to constantly balance medications. Today she works hard on taking care of her health through juicing and a healthy diet.

After her treatment finished, Nina got back to normal life, attending her regular check-ups every six months. While waiting in the doctor's rooms for the results, Nina would get a sudden "spike of anxiety." Everything was clear for several years until early 2017 when a golf ball size cyst was detected on her ovary. This involved another surgery and recovery period. I asked Nina what she has learned from her journey:

"I'm not afraid of dying. What I'm afraid of is leaving my family behind. And that's the biggest fear I had. If something happened to me, how would that impact my children? So, I wrote letters to my children, I wrote messages, I wrote journals. I didn't care what the doctors did to me, I just wanted my babies to be okay."

Throughout her treatment, the one thing Nina did not have to worry about was loss of income. She had income protection insurance in place that allowed her the time she needed to heal.

Today she is forging ahead with her career and education. Nina is a 2018 Scholarship Recipient of the Women in Leadership Executive Program. She is maintaining her health, and her family is thriving.

"If I can get through this, I can do anything."

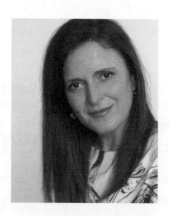

13

BOB

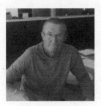

DIAGNOSIS: MELANOMA, CHILD LEUKAEMIA

Bob and his wife Rhonda are living the retirement dream. Active and fit, their home is a few steps from one of the South Coast's most beautiful beaches. They enjoy travel, exercise and time with their children and grandchildren. The day we met, Bob, aged 72, had just returned from a weekend canyoning adventure with two friends.

The road to this idyllic lifestyle presented two major health challenges which Bob and Rhonda handled in an entirely pragmatic way. As they shared their story, I was impressed by their calm, step-by-step approach to working through these life-threatening illnesses.

Bob and Rhonda's first encounter with cancer occurred 40 years ago. At that time, they had two daughters, Chris aged seven, and Jackie aged three. Rhonda regularly took them to the local swimming pool for lessons and, on this particular day, she noticed that Jackie was swimming well, but Chris got out of the pool shivering and shaking, something that was completely out of character.

They took Chris to the doctor and during her blood test, Chris' arm became horribly swollen.

Chris was well enough to go to school the next day, however midmorning, Rhonda received a phone call from their doctor who had arranged an urgent specialist appointment for Chris that afternoon. Rhonda picked up the two girls from school and Chris was admitted to hospital that day.

Chris was diagnosed with leukaemia and was set up with a regime of chemotherapy in three weekly cycles. Bob and Rhonda lived in Engadine, an outer suburb of Sydney and over an hour's drive to the Prince of Wales Hospital where Chris had her treatment. The routine of their life was turned upside down as they trekked back and forth to the hospital.

To complicate matters further, at the time when Chris was initially diagnosed, Rhonda discovered she was pregnant with their third daughter, Kim. Within months she had a newborn baby, a toddler, and a child undergoing cancer treatment.

"It was difficult to manage," recalls Rhonda. "But when you are faced with that situation, you just do what you have to do and keep going. Husbands don't stop going to work, they have to keep on going to pay for everything, so I had to do that all on my own. It was just one of those times."

Chris had chemotherapy for two years, and Rhonda admits that it was "a nightmare, going back and forth year after year, with one child undergoing chemo, another tiny tot and then a new baby."

As well as chemotherapy, Chris had radiation. They shaved her head and lines were drawn to correctly position her in the radiation machine. Forty years ago, cancer therapy was not as advanced as it is today. Bob and Rhonda remember the exhausting impact on Chris, causing her to sleep for most of the first few months of treatment.

Even though Chris handled the chemotherapy, she skipped school for a few months because her immunity was extremely low, and doctors advised she stay at home to avoid infection.

They need not have worried as all three girls have grown into adult women with fulfilling lives. Chris originally studied nursing, perhaps, they think, as a result of all the time she spent in hospital. Today Chris is 47 years old and doing very well, married and living in Brisbane. Despite warnings that she was unlikely to conceive children due to the chemotherapy drugs she was subjected to as a child, Chris has defied predictions and has two healthy children.

When cancer entered their lives again, this time it affected Bob. He had enjoyed a fulfilling career as part of a rescue helicopter crew, and later became an emergency procedures instructor for a major airline. He also spent a lot of time at the beach as a surf lifesaver. Bob has dedicated his life to the service of others and, in particular, service when people are in crisis.

In 2010, at age 64, Bob noticed a mole on his face, just next to his nose and quite close to his left eye. He wasn't too concerned, because he had always had moles; it seemed to be a hereditary condition as his mother and members of her side of the family had had a few moles, none of which were ever a problem.

This particular mole had existed for a long time but it had begun to darken. Bob's GP referred him to a specialist who examined it and offered a number of solutions: burn it off, cut it off, or just leave it and it should be fine. Bob did not really want any cutting or burning near his eye, so he thought "as long as it's not a problem, I'll put up with it."

A few months later, it was getting worse, so Bob decided to see a different specialist. As he had spent a lot of time at the beach and in the sun, Bob was aware that he was a potential melanoma candidate.

It was now around six months on from his first specialist visit. The opinion of the second specialist was that he should cut it out which he did. He advised Bob that there was unlikely to be any further problems, but just to make sure, he would send a sample off for testing.

Two days later, a phone call from that specialist confirmed that Bob had cancer. He was referred to the Melanoma Institute in Sydney. Bob believes the incredible team of doctors there saved his life. I asked Bob if he could remember how he felt when he was when first diagnosed:

"It was a bit of a shock, I suppose. People with cancer didn't seem to live that long, even the ones that you think have beaten it. I didn't think I would be around for much longer. I thought that was going to be it. I mean, I wasn't young, so I wasn't terribly worried about it. I didn't want to die, but I'd had a fairly good life, I was retired and pretty happy. I think I adjusted to it fairly alright."

The way Bob processed his diagnosis is indicative of how his career training and life experiences have shaped his thinking. As he shared his story with me, Bob projected a level-headed calmness and clear mind, the qualities of someone who has successfully dealt with emergencies and helped save and rescue others who have found themselves in life-threatening situations.

Bob took the diagnosis in his stride. The next step was a further biopsy to see how far the cancer had progressed. Unfortunately, it had reached his lymph nodes, and immediate surgery was scheduled. Bob underwent a radical neck dissection on his left side. The surgeon also performed a left superficial parotidectomy, and a wide local excision of his left cheek to remove the melanoma.

This was followed by further operations and, over the course of his journey, Bob had all the lymph nodes in his neck removed. A skin graft has skilfully restored his good looks and I could hardly tell that Bob had a scar. Unfortunately, the surgery has left Bob with a loss of sensation in that area because many nerves were removed as well. He jokes that he has to be careful not to cut himself while shaving.

Subsequent to surgery, Bob began an oral chemotherapy treatment, attending hospital every two weeks to check on his progress. As the hospital was located two hours by car or train from their home, it was quite a lot of travel to complete in a day. So rather than thinking about the check-up as a chore, Bob and Rhonda decided to treat it like a mid-week getaway, staying overnight and enjoying the sights of Sydney.

After four months of treatment, scans showed that the oral medication was causing high levels of toxicity in Bob's liver. The same medication also made Bob extremely sun sensitive, and he was not happy with being stuck indoors all the time because of his inability to cope with sunlight.

Around the same time, Bob had a routine CT scan indicating that the cancer had spread to his lungs and liver. Bob's doctors referred him on to the Westmead Melanoma Program where his medication was changed. This new drug proved effective and, over the next six months, his tumours started shrinking and then plateaued; they were still there, but not growing.

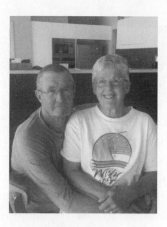

Bob and Rhonda

These were good results, and with his condition stable, Bob and Rhonda started to think about getting on with the activities they had planned for their retirement. Travel was number one on their list, and as Bob had worked for QANTAS, they wanted to take advantage of his ability to access cheaper airfares.

Bob still required treatments every three weeks, so they worked around his schedule and managed a six-week trip to Cairns with Bob flying home for treatment at the midway point and then flying back to finish the trip. They also purchased a camper trailer and had a wonderful time doing short trips all over Australia.

"We just had to make it work, there was no use being miserable."

With treatment going well, Bob's doctors gave him an extension between check-ups and they booked an overseas holiday for March 2013. Armed with all the medication Bob needed, they set off on their dream trip to Europe.

A couple of hours into the long-haul flight, Bob started shaking and sweating. He was extremely tired, and his temperature skyrocketed. The moment they disembarked, Rhonda was on the phone to Bob's doctors back in Sydney and they advised that he cease his medication.

Rhonda recounts the story of how she handled the situation—it was one of those stories that is awful at the time, but in hindsight, makes for great dinner party conversation! Bob is much taller than Rhonda and, once the plane landed at their destination airport of Frankfurt, Rhonda struggled with getting her staggering, dizzy husband off the plane and through the airport. Onlookers thought that Bob was a drunk and Rhonda was too embarrassed to ask for help, so she struggled on with Bob, got him and their luggage in a taxi and finally made it to their hotel. Fortunately, Bob recovered. He recommenced his medication, and they enjoyed the rest of their holiday.

Upon their return, Bob resumed his normal treatment and check-up schedule. A routine lung scan revealed blood clots in his lungs, adding another medication to his regime. Bob had to have daily Clexane injections for six months while being closely monitored by Westmead Hospital Clinic.

In January 2014, Bob was invited to participate in a new drug trial. This required infusions every three weeks at Westmead Hospital in Sydney. Again, they made the most of the trip, leaving early in the morning and arriving at 8am. Bob would have his blood test and a CT scan, see the doctor, then check into Casuarina Lodge, the accommodation provided at the hospital. Then if Bob felt up to it and they had enough time, they would do a little sightseeing, enjoying ferry rides to Manly or Parramatta. The following day Bob would have his infusion treatment and then they would head home.

This cycle continued for two years with 35 cycles of treatment. Bob's melanomas responded and today, two years after his last treatment, Bob is doing very well, and his check-ups are now spaced at six months, rather than three months.

Throughout Bob's journey, Rhonda has been a great support. I have so much admiration for her role in taking care of both Chris and Bob, while raising their family. She is an extremely positive person, and I feel that Bob and Rhonda work well together as a team.

I asked Bob if he had any regrets, anything he would have done differently. The only thing he wonders is what would have happened if he had removed the mole on his first visit to the specialist. Perhaps it might not have progressed to his lymph nodes and he would not have had to go through extreme surgery and treatment to save his life. Bob is philosophical about the past, he is not one to live with regret about something he cannot change:

"So, it's just the way life happens. I could have walked out the door and got hit by a car."

Now Bob is 72, and one of the main things that has kept him active is his love of canyoning. Rhonda jokingly tells me about Bob's '200 Club' where he and his "stupid mates" go on canyoning trips three or four times a year. Why the 200 Club? Their ages add up to 200! Rhonda attributes these trips and Bob's enthusiasm for planning them as a key factor in his positive outlook and recovery.

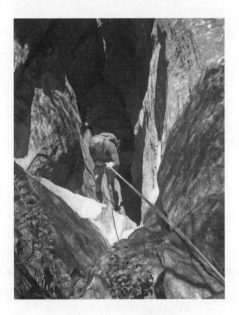

Bob on a canyoning adventure

Bob and Rhonda continue to thrive because they have active routines and always look forward. They wake up every morning and go swimming and take walks. They get in their camper trailer and go for driving holidays. They go on overseas trips and have just returned from a visit to Israel, Egypt and Jordan. They make plans for the future and live life to the full.

"You've got to have a purpose."

14

HELEN

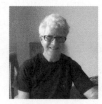

Diagnosis: Breast Cancer

Helen is a softly spoken woman with a caring heart for others. At 74, she is super active, happy and healthy with a passion for dragon boat racing.

Helen's diagnosis and treatment occurred in 1992, many years before there was widespread awareness and fundraising for breast cancer. Her journey is not only notable for the good health she currently enjoys, but also because it provided the impetus for Helen to dedicate her life to supporting other women with breast cancer.

A primary school teacher for many years, Helen balanced her career with raising two children. Eddie, Helen's husband, is an exuberant Yorkshireman and the pair embody the adage that opposites attract. Helen admits that she used to internalise her thoughts, happy to let Eddie do all the talking, but she is now learning to "get things out" and be more communicative.

When Helen was just 48-years old, she noticed a lump in her right breast. She was fairly unconcerned because 12 years prior, Helen had found a similar lump and, in that instance, it was removed and confirmed as benign. Apart from that experience, Helen felt that her fitness level and active lifestyle made her an unlikely candidate for any type of illness.

The new lump was not painful, but she decided to have it checked by her GP. A mammogram and ultrasound test followed, and Helen was told that everything was okay.

A short time later, Helen noticed that her breast was starting to change shape. Despite reassurance from her doctor she instinctively felt there was something wrong.

"Be aware of your body and any changes in your skin, not just your breasts, and even when the test results don't show up anything, if you have a feeling that it's not right, then persist."

Helen booked another appointment with her GP. As her usual doctor was away, Helen saw a different doctor and asked for a referral to see the surgeon she had seen previously.

The surgeon looked at her breast and told her that the lump had to come out. There was no biopsy, Helen was booked straight into hospital for surgery the following week. She was in hospital for nine days, and her recovery was slower than expected. She felt quite emotional and decided not to return to work until after the stitches were removed.

Following surgery, Helen was asked to come back in for the results. Eddie was supposed to be at work that day, but she asked him to accompany her to the appointment.

"As soon as we arrived, the doctor beckoned us into his office so we both kind of knew it was something serious. He said that I had to have the whole breast off. I didn't even know what a mastectomy was, people didn't talk about it back then."

Helen was informed that she had to have a right modified radical mastectomy and she remembers being more terrified of the word 'radical' than the word 'cancer.' Upon hearing the news, Helen just felt numb.

"I didn't really understand what was happening. Eddie was the same and he got lost driving me back home, we just both couldn't take it in. Eddie went back to work, he's the type of person who talks everything out. The people at work said, 'You've got her dead and buried already...my mother had breast cancer and she's still alive at 80.' When you hear stories like that, it helps you."

Unlike today, there were no breast cancer awareness campaigns. Helen did not know anyone else who had been through the experience. Eddie tried to research what he could and back then, the only place to find information was at the library.

Helen had the mastectomy and according to her surgeon, it was an absolute success and no further treatment was required. As Helen shared this part of the story, she laughed. She now finds it amusing that she actually believed him, when nothing could have been further from the truth!

Two of the lymph nodes removed proved to be cancerous, and Helen needed to have both radiation and chemotherapy. She was immediately prescribed Tamoxifen, which caused her to experience early menopause.

Helen started treatment with radiation therapy for five weeks which she handled quite well. After that she was sent to the oncologist and burst into tears because she was so scared of the drugs going into her body. Due to her low white cell count, Helen's chemotherapy was set at intervals of four weeks instead of three weeks over a period of six months. As for side-effects, she suffered lymphoedema in her arm, but overall Helen feels lucky that she coped quite well.

At the end of her treatments, Helen faced what she felt was perhaps the most dreadful moment of her journey. Her doctor said he did not need to see her anymore.

"I felt lost. Who was going to look after me now? I had put the onus on someone else to look after me rather than doing it myself. I felt safe while I was under his care and having regular checks."

It was not until this final appointment that Helen asked for some documentation and to be informed of the exact type of cancer she had. He told her it was an aggressive Stage 3 cancer. This surprised Helen, because all along she still had the feeling that maybe they had made a mistake.

Eddie was Helen's main support throughout her surgeries and treatment. At the time of her diagnosis, Helen's son was away in Canada and her daughter was living in New Zealand, but they both came home to be with their mother. This was wonderful, but Helen regrets not being transparent about her condition. If she had been honest about how she felt, it would have fostered greater understanding and allowed them to provide better support.

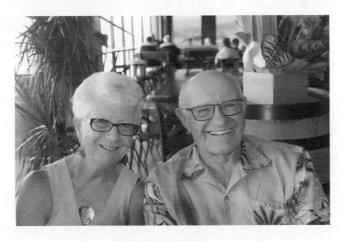

Helen and Eddie

"I needed to communicate more. I don't know if it would have made a difference, but it would have helped when I wasn't feeling the best. Eddie would ask, 'How do you feel today?' I would say 'alright,' even when I wasn't because I didn't want to worry him. Whereas if Eddie's got something wrong, I will know all about it!"

Her sisters and brothers were also supportive, but they were shocked when they heard Helen's diagnosis as she was the one amongst them who ran, swam, ate well and lived a healthy lifestyle. Keen to restore her good health and rebuild her strength, Helen took back control of her own wellbeing. She had always been an exercise freak and became even more so with a program of swimming, walking and going to the gym. The other area she and Eddie investigated was natural therapies and a holistic approach to healing and living.

A naturopath put Helen on a supplement regime and she truly believes they have helped her recovery. Helen did find it amusing that when she went back to see her original GP and asked if there were any vitamins she could take to build herself up, he was a little embarrassed that he had dismissed her concerns and told her to take a multivitamin!

Eddie and Helen have also incorporated other therapies to improve their quality of life, including regular chiropractic adjustments, aromatherapy sessions, massages and tai chi classes.

The other element that helped Helen's psychological wellbeing was a local support group run by a breast care nurse who provided helpful information about how to deal with the after-effects of breast cancer. Most importantly, the group connected Helen with other women who had been through similar journeys.

Helen went back to work and continued teaching, talking about her experience to everyone she knew. The awareness of her diagnosis resulted in many women having mammograms. She became such an advocate that she was asked to volunteer to mentor breast cancer patients in hospital. Helen also became one of the first women to volunteer at her local breast screening clinic. On the days when women would be called back for additional testing, Helen would be there to provide support.

The lack of information available for her journey motivated Helen to do more. When the BCNA began in 1998, Helen worked closely with them to create an information kit that is now available to every Australian woman who is diagnosed with breast cancer. She is often asked to speak at events and strongly urges women to seek support from the BCNA and to get their My Journey Kit.

After 38 years of teaching, Helen retired. She went through a period of depression and looking back, she thinks the trigger may have been a combination of things, but the main reason was leaving work and, "feeling like she was of no use anymore."

This all changed for Helen when she became involved in Breast

Cancer Survivor Dragon Boat Racing, a concept that was initially started by Canadian sports medicine specialist Don McKenzie and is now an international movement. Dragon boat paddling is proven to assist with regaining upper body mobility and reducing lymphoedema after breast cancer.

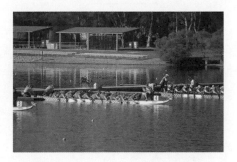

Helen in action, dragon boat racing

When Helen's support group formed the Dragons Abreast team, they trained together and went on to compete in their first regatta in Canada. Helen has been the president of her local dragon boat club for the past three years. On the day we met, I saw a lovely floral arrangement on her table. Helen had decided to step down as president and the flowers were a thank you gift in recognition of her service.

"I needed to learn to say no, I'm not doing it anymore. I'll still be involved, but I'm learning to prioritise. Maybe that's one of the lessons that cancer teaches us...not to be martyrs."

Helen credits breast cancer with helping her grow as a person. She continues to help other women on their journeys and her past 26 years of good health is a shining example that there is life after breast cancer.

"Life didn't go back to normal, whatever that is, and I was determined to make it better. I learnt to stress less and make the most of every day. I also worked hard to stop hiding my thoughts and tried to speak my mind more often instead of trying to please everyone."

15

KEN AND DEBBIE

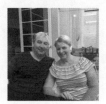

DIAGNOSIS: NON-HODGKIN'S LYMPHOMA/BREAST CANCER

Ken and Debbie have been firm friends of mine for more than 10 years. Ken is, without doubt, the most pragmatic man I have ever met. He has that wonderful ability to see things clearly and does not "sweat the small stuff." Debbie is his match: she too sees the practical side of things and yet has the caring and compassionate qualities that make her a cherished friend.

KEN

I met them when Ken, the business entrepreneur, was looking for a copywriter. He has operated many different types of businesses over his lifetime from car dealerships and horse training enterprises through to innovative video production and technology companies. Even though he is now 67, I cannot imagine him taking the traditional retirement route as he is always working on some kind of interesting project.

After a few years working overseas, Ken and Debbie decided to return to Australia in 2004. Ken was 53 at the time and recalls noticing a lump under his arm as they were preparing for the move.

He self-diagnosed that it was not serious and decided to have it looked at once he settled on the Gold Coast in Queensland, Australia.

I was horrified when Ken described the lump as being the size of a tennis ball and asked him how he managed to hide it from Debbie for such a long time. "Simple," he replied. "I just kept my arm down."

When Ken finally went to his local GP, I sense that his doctor had the same reaction as me, immediately referring Ken to a surgeon who took one look and booked him in for surgery within 48 hours.

Ken went home from that appointment, not stressed or shocked about the diagnosis, but instead feeling uneasy about the recommended treatment. He knew that there was an issue that had to be dealt with, but the rushed surgery just did not sit right with him.

"I thought, 'Why wouldn't we have a look and confirm exactly what it is first?' Then, I thought, 'No, trust my gut.' I went back to him and said, 'I'm not going to do that, I want another opinion.'"

Many people have told me that they felt coerced into one form of treatment or another. The important thing to remember is that you have the right to decide what happens to your body. Ken exercised his right to choose and credits his decision to get a second opinion as the reason he is still alive today.

Debbie started researching lymphoma and the different types of treatment available. She came to the conclusion that cutting into this type of cancer could dramatically increase its chance of spreading.

They went to the hospital and another doctor examined his symptoms. Without any tests, Ken was told that he had cancer and he was going to die. He took this information with a grain of salt as he had not yet had a biopsy.

Ken had the biopsy on his birthday and he remembers them taking "a few chunks out of it." He also had a scan which showed a band of 13 tumours from the size of a tennis ball in his armpit, gradually decreasing to the size of a marble inside his body.

The doctors finally confirmed a diagnosis of Follicular Lymphoma, a slow growing cancer that he had ignored for a long time. Ken was very pleased with his decision not to have surgery, as this would not have solved his problem and could have exacerbated it.

Ken's oncologist started him on CHOP, the acronym for his chemotherapy regimen. Every three weeks for nine months, Ken attended oncology for his infusion and treatment. The first two days after treatment he would feel good due to the steroid Prednisone, then his energy would drop off before slowly building up again before the next cycle would begin.

The main side-effects that Ken suffered were baldness, extreme tiredness and a lack of sleep. He found that he was up all night and fortuitously surprised a burglar off on one occasion.

"I got through it. I never really noticed, other than the fact that I was bald as a badger; I lost every hair on my body and I felt off sometimes. I thought, just get on with it."

After his nine months of treatment, Ken had regular blood tests to check on his status, but the bloods did not tell the full story. Four years later in 2008, new lumps appeared. This time, he knew exactly what was happening.

By that time, a new drug called Rituximab, branded MabThera, was developed and Ken was treated with this drug twice weekly for around four months. For Ken, the MabThera had no side-effects and for the next nine years he felt "like brand new."

All was well until Ken noticed a persistent cough. A PET scan just before Christmas 2017 showed that lymphoma had returned in his throat, groin and lungs. Ken is back on MabThera and chemotherapy and he is as positive as ever about his outcome.

"I think that a lot of people worry themselves to death with cancer, but at the end of the day, what can you do about it? Nothing so just get on with it. It's just like a headache, take your medicine and keep moving. That's basically my motto."

DEBBIE

As a young New Zealand woman, Debbie led a fascinating life and her name will forever be in the horse racing history books. In a world dominated by men, it was not until 1977 that the New Zealand Racing Conference finally approved the licensing of women riders and Debbie was amongst the first group of female jockeys in her home country, riding many winners.

The highlight of Debbie's career was her 1982 ride on Deb's Mate at The Cox Plate, one of the most prestigious events on the Australian racing calendar. She was the first female jockey to ever ride in this event, paving the way for all the female jockeys in the sport today.

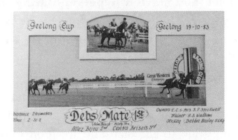

Debbie's win on Deb's Mate at the Geelong Cup

Since her racing days, Debbie's skill with people has led her to customer service roles in the produce, travel and banking industries. She has worked in a number of interesting roles, while travelling often and socialising regularly with friends and family.

In 2013, at age 52, Debbie found a small lump in her right breast and ignored it for a week or two hoping it would go away, but it remained the same. After what she had already been through with Ken, Debbie decided to book herself in for a mammogram.

When she arrived at the clinic, she was asked if she had a lump. Debbie was told that if she said 'yes', they could not go ahead with the mammogram, telling her that she would have to go and see her GP. Debbie found the situation quite confusing and ended up saying 'no', so that they would go ahead with the screening.

She considers herself lucky that she had the mammogram as two weeks later she was called back for an ultrasound. When she arrived for the appointment, Debbie was informed that she would actually be having a biopsy, which was unsettling as she was not expecting an invasive procedure. Debbie went ahead with the biopsy, and told me that even at that stage, she was not worried about the outcome.

"I was one of those people that thought this happened to other people, not me. This will be nothing. I honestly thought it would be nothing."

Debbie took Ken with her to hear the results and remembers sitting down and being told she had breast cancer.

"I was in shock and started hyperventilating. Ken just sat there looking at me, he didn't even put his arm around me, and the doctor ended up comforting me. We were both just in shock."

Everything from this point on moved very quickly. Debbie was booked in to see a surgeon who recommended a mastectomy rather than a lumpectomy due to the size and location of the lump, being quite close to the nipple. She recalls the stress of having to make an instant decision between these two procedures while the surgeon, a registrar and three student doctors stood there waiting. Debbie did not have the time or space to process what had been said but felt pressured to answer so she agreed to the mastectomy of her right breast and was promptly booked in for surgery the following week.

Debbie walked out of that appointment feeling rushed and not able to properly consider her options. In hindsight she realises that she was in shock and even if she could have asked questions, she would not have known what to ask at that consultation.

"I just wish that he had said to us, do you want to go away for half an hour, have a coffee, sit down and discuss it and then come back and tell me your decision."

As they left the surgeon's rooms, Debbie told Ken that she thought she would prefer to have a double mastectomy rather than living with just one breast. When they arrived home, Debbie phoned the surgeon's office and made her request. She was told that she would need to come in for another appointment to discuss it with the doctor.

"He asked me why I would want to do that. I said, 'I just don't want to live with the worry that it can come back.' He said it was unlikely. I told him that was fine to say, but I would be the one living with it, so I said, 'No, I've made the decision to have both off, I'd rather live with none than one. I would feel weird.'"

The surgery was successful, and Debbie only took six weeks off work. She was employed as a casual and if she did not work, she did not get paid, so she went back as soon as she could. Fortunately, her recovery went well and by about three months, she began to feel normal again.

Chemotherapy began once her wounds were healed. She had treatment in three weekly cycles for six months. The first two cycles were tolerable, but by the third cycle, Debbie was lying in bed not wanting to move because everything hurt.

"Even my eyelashes hurt. I said to myself, 'I'm never going through this again ever. If it comes back, I'm never doing chemo. It was just horrible, the worst days of my life.'"

A year on, doctors recommended that Debbie have her ovaries and tubes removed due to a high risk of contracting ovarian cancer. Debbie tells me that she really did not want to have this done and she kept saying 'no', but it was friends and family who kept insisting. She eventually gave in and had them removed.

As with most breast cancer patients, Debbie was prescribed the drug Tamoxifen for five years. This caused a range of side-effects including dizziness and hot flushes. The worst effect was aching bones and joints. After two years, she chose to stop taking the medication, as the pain was unbearable.

Debbie expressed that friends and family were very supportive, "Even Ken," she said with a tongue-in-cheek laugh. She found that most people were not too intrusive, and I pointed out that Ken probably kept them at bay!

After three years of living without breasts and the subsequent removal of her ovaries and tubes, Debbie started to think about reconstruction. At the time of her mastectomy, she did not really consider it, but three years on, her feelings were changing.

"I didn't even feel like a female, I just felt like a body. I was sick of wearing men's t-shirts because they were the only ones that fit because they are made for a flat chest. And I would see other women out there wearing nice tops and dresses and I would think 'I couldn't wear that because I would look ridiculous.'"

Debbie began researching her options, deciding against implants as she knew a few ladies who had experienced problems with them. She chose to have a DIEP Flap reconstruction where the fat, skin and blood vessels are cut from the wall of the lower belly and moved up to the chest to rebuild the breasts.

It was a ten-hour surgery involving two surgeons and overall, was very successful. She is very happy with the results and thrilled to have her belly disappear and put to great use!

Ken and Debbie are happy and enjoying life. It is always great to see them, and our catch-ups are inevitably peppered with Ken's dry one liners and stories from their latest cruise!

"Seeing Ken go through cancer and coming through it made it a bit easier for me. If you haven't witnessed it yourself, it's easy to believe all the horror stories you read."

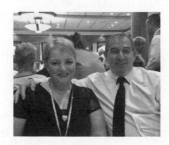

16

REX

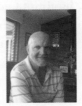

DIAGNOSIS: PROSTATE CANCER

When Rex was diagnosed with prostate cancer on April Fool's Day, he thought it must be a joke. His unique reaction requires context: this is a man who had me laughing from the moment I met him—Rex quite accurately likens himself to English comic John Cleese and my mind immediately conjures up the TV Series Fawlty Towers.

The more pertinent reason for Rex's disbelief was that he is a fit and healthy man with an active lifestyle and a totally positive outlook on life. Rex describes himself as "bulletproof," never imagining for a moment that anything could hold him back from his dynamic life.

As a teacher for 37 years, he worked in an environment where he developed great rapport with students, peers and parents. I can imagine he was a favourite teacher who ensured his students thrived through captivating learning methods.

Rex retired at age 56, to start an exciting new phase of his life with time to travel, play with his grandchildren, and enjoy social adventures with good friends.

It was a routine blood test at age 60 that alerted Rex's GP to the possibility of prostate cancer. His prostate-specific antigen (PSA) level was slightly elevated, so his doctor asked him to return in three months to repeat the test. Rex had no other symptoms and continued to keep busy.

Three months later, the follow-up blood test showed his PSA levels were extremely elevated and Rex was sent directly to a urologist who arranged further scans and tests.

"I had every test, all the scans and I think that was more draining than anything, having to go in and wait, do fasting and all that kind of stuff. It was frustrating because I just wanted to get it all out of the way and get on with the rest of my life."

After his biopsy, Rex was asked to donate his sample to medical research and he was more than happy to do so, hoping it would help someone in the future. At the time, he was told that the current statistics for probability of prostate cancer were 60% for men aged in their sixties, 70% for men in their seventies and 80% for men aged upwards from eighty.

Rex went back to the urologist for the results on that fateful April Fool's day with his wife Helen. They expected there would be some health issue, but Rex remained positive. The urologist told them he definitely had prostate cancer, and that it was very aggressive. Rex immediately asked about his prognosis, explaining, "I'm the type of person who wants to know," and his doctor bluntly said he had six months to live.

Helen was a bit shocked at the news, but Rex saw it as something he would deal with and overcome.

"I felt positive at the diagnosis because I had had such a good life. I'm not the type of person that goes into depression, not very often, everyone gets depressed sometimes, but I get over it very quickly and I thought, 'No, this is unfortunate that I've got this problem.' So, I worked on changing my lifestyle, cutting down on my alcohol to get ready for the operation. I felt that if I got fit and healthy, I could deal with it."

Prior to surgery, Rex was sent to the physiotherapist to learn some exercises to minimise the effects of the surgery. She told him to expect some incontinence, even for a short while, and made a joke that if he laughed too hard or farted, he would probably leak!

The surgery was actually the easiest part for Rex. The doctors had warned him that they would not know how far the cancer had spread and whether or not it had escaped the prostate until they actually performed the surgery. As it turned out, Rex had a quick two-hour operation and three hours later he was dressed and discharged. His surgeon reported that due to Rex's fitness and low body fat, the operation was one of the easiest he had ever done.

Performed using the Da Vinci surgical system, Rex had a robotic prostatectomy which was minimally invasive, entering via the belly button and down through the penis to remove the prostate. Rex recovered remarkably well. It was a very successful surgery, fortunately not requiring any further intervention as the cancer had not progressed outside the prostate.

Rex even impressed his physiotherapist when he informed her that he had full bladder control. She was amazed, and Rex joked that he was relieved that he did not have to wear nappies!

Sent home with orders to rest for six weeks, Rex admits he ignored these instructions and was "naughty." From the outside, Rex looked fine. There were no large surgical incisions to heal, so Rex assumed he was well enough to go back to his normal life. Helen was very supportive but found it impossible to get her patient to rest when he insisted on going at his usual pace.

During his recovery period, Rex and Helen's daughter and son-in-law were adding an extension to their house, and naturally Rex offered to lend a hand. He was carrying earth and mortar and getting stuck into the work. In hindsight, he feels that he may have done some damage; it is impossible to know if he did, but at the time, he felt well able to do it.

Due to the success of Rex's surgery, he was told that he had a 75% chance of regaining erectile function.

"It never happened, so that's just the way it is. That's the luck of the draw. And that was the worst part for me. It hit

me like a ton of bricks. I'd lost my manhood and that took a lot for me to come to terms with. It was the biggest shock. I had to deal with not feeling like a man anymore and that was the hardest thing for me to accept."

Doctors advised that it could take up to two years to restore erectile function. As Rex was still only 61, he explored different medications, but the side effects were awful, giving him weird dreams, and a foggy, fuzzy head. It made him lethargic, and it also affected his ability to drive a car, so he decided to stop taking it. After this experience, Rex and Helen decided not to pursue other medication avenues.

It is now six years on, and I ask Rex if this disappointment still affects him. His response is a message to all of us when tragedy strikes. It is a reminder not to dwell on the bad, but to be grateful for all the good we have in our lives: Rex says he is thankful that they got all the cancer; he is happy to be alive; and thrilled to be fit and healthy enough to play with his grandchildren.

Rex goes back every year for a check-up and shakes as he worries about what the results will be, but for the last six years he has been all clear and continues to view each day as a bonus. He attributes a lot of this to his daughter who attends seminars and researches healthy eating and living. She advised Rex and Helen about the benefits of sourcing organic fresh foods from farmers' markets, eating natural wholefoods and minimising radiation from electronic devices and wiring.

One person who helped Rex through the emotional and mental aspects was his brother-in-law, a fellow prostate cancer survivor.

"He's a great guy, and talking to him really helped me, he was very supportive. He would come over and we would talk about how he dealt with the emotional side of things."

Rex realises that not everyone has someone like this in their family for support and recommends that anyone who finds themselves in this situation goes to a men's group. He believes that meeting other men who have been through the same journey is one of the best ways to deal with the effects of prostate cancer.

Perhaps it is from his teaching days, but Rex feels strongly about the importance of finding a mentor, someone you can talk to freely, someone who will listen and encourage you. Rex found a mentor in his neighbour, a man who shared his wisdom and today Rex continues paying it forward by mentoring students.

Known as an excellent teacher, Rex is often asked to help out with tutoring children from foster families or children who are having discipline or learning difficulties at school. He tells me just a few stories of the children he has worked with, and I cannot help but think that this is his calling. He talks about one particular eight-year-old boy whose behaviour was appalling and his parents had given up any hope of improvement. When Rex started tutoring the boy, he was rude, petulant and swore constantly making it impossible to actually do any teaching. Rex used techniques and knowledge honed over his teaching career and today the boy is a well behaved 14-year-old who is forever thankful for the difference Rex made in his life.

Rex makes sure every day is a good day. No matter where he is, or who he is with, at the dinner table every evening he asks each person, "What's been the best part of your day?"

It is such a simple, yet powerful question that no matter how annoyed or grumpy you feel, it insists that you think of something positive so that you focus on the good in your life. Rex is inspiring everyone around him every day, and on the day that I met him, hearing his story was definitely the best part of my day.

"Mentoring someone who is going through what you have been through is a powerful form of support."

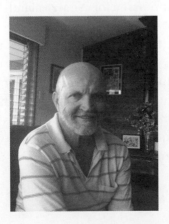

17

SHARON

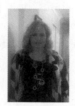

DIAGNOSIS: CLEAR CELL CARCINOMA OF THE CERVIX

Travel is in Sharon's DNA. As a young girl growing up in Cape Town, South Africa, Sharon always wanted to travel and at the age of 24, she left on the adventure of a lifetime with nothing more than a backpack, a sleeping bag and a copy of Lonely Planet. She explored the UK, Europe and the Middle East before meeting and marrying a New Zealander. They travelled together throughout South East Asia on their way to settle permanently in the "Land of the Long White Cloud" (a translation of the Maori name for New Zealand).

Sharon was born with a condition that she did not discover until she was 19 years old. It is not unusual for a girl to get the odd urinary tract infection (UTI), but Sharon was getting them frequently. One time it was so bad that she could not get out of bed and the doctor made a house call that led to him taking her to hospital in his own car. Sharon was immediately admitted, and this was the beginning of two difficult years of being in and out of hospital with multiple bladder, kidney and urinary tract infections caused by a condition known as Vesicoureteral reflux.

After the problem was eventually diagnosed, Sharon was treated with medication and advised that, due to her condition, she could not have children. The symptoms did settle down and a few years later she set off on her trip overseas.

Sharon was 25 when she settled in Auckland, New Zealand and decided to turn her love of travel into a career by studying Business Management and Tourism at the Auckland University of Technology. One day she was feeling unwell and went to her doctor who discovered she was pregnant, Unfortunately, she was having a miscarriage, and the doctor was concerned about her blood pressure. That is when her kidney problems resurfaced.

"I was a bit taken aback by it all. They asked me to have an ultrasound and midway through the procedure, the sonographer excused herself from the room and returned with all these doctors."

The ultrasound had revealed that Sharon's right kidney was virtually destroyed and her left kidney was enlarged. After further testing, her right kidney was below acceptable levels and Sharon was advised that it was better to live with one functioning kidney than dealing with the strain of the failed kidney.

Sharon was scheduled for surgery through the public health system which meant waiting five long months during which time she attended doctors' appointments, frequent hospital visits, and took numerous medications to keep her well for the operation.

At this point Sharon was aged 32 and had finished her studies. Even though her body needed the surgery, Sharon was not emotionally prepared for what was to happen.

"I went into denial. I didn't want to know, I didn't want to hear about it. But I knew I had to have it done and just wanted it over and done with."

Her reticence continued once she arrived at the hospital.

"I didn't want to go into the room to prepare myself for the operation. I didn't want to lie down, I was emotionally

fighting the whole way. It's not that I'm an obstructive person, or someone that would deliberately challenge anybody. I think it was more the denial because to me, I didn't feel sick."

Sharon eventually walked herself into the operating theatre and gave in to the process and allowed the doctor to perform a nephrectomy. Her recovery was slow, taking months rather than weeks because her body was not eliminating the toxins from her body due to the reflux. This made her whole system sluggish and hindered healing.

"The thing I found the hardest was the drugs. The morphine and the epidural were horrendous. They made me very sick and the recovery process was awful."

For Sharon, it was a vicious cycle—she needed the medications for pain relief and to prevent infection, however her compromised kidneys and gut had difficulty processing them. Sharon feels that the side effects from the drugs caused as big an impact as the actual surgery. With the help of her Mum, who flew over from South Africa to look after her, Sharon gradually improved.

Two years after the operation, Sharon discovered she was pregnant. It was news that she processed with mixed feelings following her earlier miscarriage and the advice from her doctor as a teenager. It was also bad timing because her relationship was not going well and, during her pregnancy, Sharon actually decided to end her relationship.

Due to her medical history, Sharon was closely monitored with multiple check-ups and medical appointments during every week of her pregnancy. The morning sickness was making her increasingly ill and, if not for her understanding boss, Sharon would not have been able to continue working. At the 26-week mark, Sharon's high-risk pregnancy reached the point when her medical team insisted on admitting her to hospital.

You have probably gathered by now that Sharon hates hospitals. Imagine her reaction when she was told to stay in hospital for the remainder of her pregnancy—Sharon was not amused. She endured for four weeks and her reward was the birth of her daughter Caitlin, who arrived at 30 weeks weighing just 1.4 kg (3 lb 2 oz). The newborn was whisked off to the Neonatal Intensive Care Unit (NICU).

"I was taken to ICU where I was given a polaroid photo of my baby. I was wheeled in my bed to the NICU at 5pm to see Caitlin for the first time. She was full of pipes and tubes and I couldn't touch her or hold her. It was another traumatic process."

At the age of 11, Caitlin was diagnosed with Asperger's Syndrome and Dyspraxia. Prior to that, the doctors advised Sharon that Caitlin's development and constant illness was probably due to her premature birth or her low birth weight, but Sharon wonders if the medication she took during her pregnancy may have also contributed. For five years Caitlin was in and out of Starship Children's Hospital with pneumonia and bronchiolitis. Despite her distressing beginnings, she is now 17 and doing very well.

Support for Sharon and Caitlin arrived in the form of Sharon's mother who travelled to Auckland and stayed for four months.

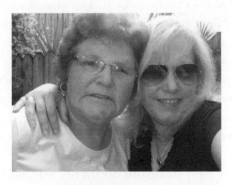

Sharon with her Mum

After her Mum left, Sharon returned to work but found that the childcare costs were extremely high. She decided to move to South Africa, but due to Caitlin's status as a New Zealander, plus the uncertain future of South Africa, they ended up returning to Auckland. Sharon was rehired by her previous employer but the instability in the

Middle East in 2003 affected the New Zealand tourism industry and she took a voluntary redundancy, using the opportunity to spend quality time with her daughter.

Sharon knew that she would eventually have to return to the workforce. Her problems were solved when her mother decided to visit and she stayed in New Zealand for 18 months so that Sharon could get back on her feet with a teaching position in tourism.

In 2006, at the age of 39, Sharon's health problems resurfaced and her GP prescribed an ongoing kidney and blood pressure medication.

"It was traumatic for me to realise that I would be on drugs for the rest of my life. I didn't like the idea of taking medication and accepting I will always have a medical condition. Eventually all those drugs start to take their toll. My gut was being affected, I was becoming reactive to antibiotics and anti-inflammatories."

The following year, Sharon was prescribed anti-inflammatory tablets. She started feeling sick, and one night took additional tablets, not realising that it was the tablets causing the problem. The following day she reached out for medical help. The closest place was a medical centre near her office in Auckland CBD so she had no alternative but to go there. This became a turning point in her medical care.

"I saw a doctor who ended up saving my life a few years later. She saw me and went through my history and took me off the anti-inflammatories and changed my blood pressure medication."

Sharon immediately made this doctor her GP. She was impressed at the pro-active way the doctor looked at her complicated medical history and grateful for her focus on improving her quality of life.

One of the first recommendations was for Sharon to stop taking the contraceptive pill and to be assessed for a tubal ligation. Sharon was deemed ineligible through the public health system, but her feisty doctor fought her case and made it happen. She also performed the pap smear that led to Sharon's Clear Cell Carcinoma diagnosis.

It was 2010 and Sharon was travelling in the South Island of New Zealand with clients when she received a call from the hospital to make an appointment that week. She was taken aback as she was still waiting for the results of her pap smear from her GP. After that call, her GP called and apologised, saying that the hospital was very proactive and that the smear results showed an abnormality that needed to be reviewed. Sharon went to the hospital for further tests—the pap smear was fine, but the vault smear showed an anomaly.

"I wasn't worried about it because I didn't believe that it could possibly be cervical cancer, I didn't fit any of the criteria. Unbeknownst to me there are various types of cancer, the cervix is just the location."

The gynaecologist rang Sharon at work and told her that she had cancer. He then said due to his unfamiliarity with the type of cancer, he would arrange a second pathology assessment of the bloods and it could take a couple of weeks.

After a worrying two weeks, her doctor confirmed she had Clear Cell Carcinoma and that she would need a radical hysterectomy. Sharon immediately fired a million questions at him, wanting to know all about it. He referred her to the leading oncologist in the country and Sharon soon discovered that she was of great interest to the entire oncology department because she was the first person in New Zealand to be diagnosed with Clear Cell Carcinoma of the cervix, an extremely rare type of cancer.

The recommended treatment was a hysterectomy. Sharon's specialist suggested that she could have her ovaries removed at the same time, but she opted to leave the decision in the hands of her oncology team by signing a document allowing them to remove the ovaries if they deemed it to be necessary. This is a decision she now regrets as she has since found out that she is in the high-risk category for ovarian cancer.

"I was very, very lucky. The cancer was seven millimetres (0.28 inch) so it had not spread to my lymph nodes. It was pure luck that we caught it in time because it is a fast

spreading cancer. I had no symptoms, by the time I got symptoms it could have been too late."

Sharon credits the speed from diagnosis to operation as a key factor in saving her life. When she compares the recovery from her hysterectomy to that of her nephrectomy, Sharon feels it was much easier and quicker because she was fitter. Prior to the hysterectomy, she was going to the gym three times a week and her doctors agree that this made the difference.

The main complication during recovery from the hysterectomy was that her mother, who had come to New Zealand to look after her, suffered a heart attack and had to have quintuple bypass surgery. The operation cost $65,000 and Sharon had to go back to work a mere four weeks after her hysterectomy to help pay for it.

"We managed it. You don't think about anything other than what you have to do to save your family. You get on with it and you survive."

Sharon held it together emotionally throughout her cancer journey and her mother's heart surgery, but after she was cleared, she suffered from anger. Sometimes it is the initial diagnosis that is the worst and for others, something else triggers their emotions.

"Once it was all over, I got angry. All these emotions built up inside me. It was like I was given a calm tablet, and then suddenly this wave of emotion came through me and that was anger and I didn't know how to deal with it. The only thing that helped me was exercise. No specialist, no psychologist, no doctor, just exercise. Going to the gym and just pushing myself. That's what got me through to the other end. To me, that is really, really important."

Today Sharon runs her own travel and tourism company and her priorities are to keep well, to look after her gut health and to keep a balance between work and health. She wants to be sure that if anything

else happens to her medically, that she is fit and well enough to deal
with it.

**"I'm proud of myself for getting through cancer. And I'm
proud of myself for getting through all the things I did.
That is the positive thing that came out of my experiences
and I focus on that."**

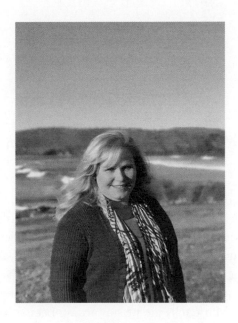

18

GRAHAM

DIAGNOSIS: PERITONEAL CANCER

I was introduced to Graham by his fabulous daughters who I have known for a few years. Over the course of our friendship, I heard that Graham had been through a rare and serious cancer. Of particular interest is the fact that Graham is a 10-year survivor and continues to thrive. I was excited to meet him for a chat.

At 67, Graham looks well, perhaps in better shape than many men his age. His wife Marie tells me he has always been a fit man, and even though he is now retired, his working life as a builder created a positive pattern of an active rather than a sedentary life.

Graham's cancer journey began with a routine hernia operation in 2009 when he was aged 57. His hernia was successfully repaired, however the doctor informed him that, while he was performing the surgery, he noticed some irregularities and took a few tissue samples for testing.

Several days later, Graham's doctor called him in to say that his appendix had burst some time ago and it needed to be removed. He was again admitted to hospital and during the appendectomy, the surgeon discovered cancer cells on the wall of the appendix. Graham was immediately referred to one of Australia's leading gastrointestinal surgeons who diagnosed him with peritoneal cancer.

A rare cancer that develops in the lining of the abdomen and on the walls of abdominal organs, peritoneal cancer is difficult to diagnose because it does not appear as a tumour in an organ. For Graham, having elective hernia surgery literally saved his life—if the doctor had not seen the abnormal cells during that initial operation, the cancer may not have been discovered until it was too late.

I asked Graham how he reacted to his diagnosis. Being a practical and logical person, he focussed on the solution rather than the problem. It sounded like a straightforward operation and he expected to be back working again in no time. The reality did not fully impact him until he arrived for the operation.

"I think it hit hard when I first got into hospital and especially when I felt how crook I was after the operation."

For Marie, the initial diagnosis affected her the most:

"When the doctor took us into the room to explain, it was just like he punched me in the stomach and I just went to tears thinking, 'Oh my god, what just happened?' And from then on, I just thought, 'This is not going to beat us.'"

Two weeks after his diagnosis, Graham was in an 11-hour surgery having a peritonectomy. His gallbladder, spleen and part of his bowel was removed along with the cancerous cells in the peritoneum.

Graham recovered initially in ICU. After five days, he was treated with HIPEC, a highly concentrated heated chemotherapy treatment that is poured directly into the abdominal cavity and heated to 42 degrees Celsius. He was rolled from side to side to allow the liquid to come in contact with all the cavity walls before it was drained out of him. This process was repeated every day for five days.

"The pain was horrendous. I was on morphine, but it still felt like I was getting my insides burnt out."

Thankfully, Graham did not need any further treatment and he could focus on recovery. It was a slow process to restore normal digestive function—he had no appetite and was constipated. For an active and driven person like Graham, the situation was frustrating.

"It was a long road back. I didn't feel like visitors and it made me a bit of a recluse."

During these early days after the operation, Graham felt like many other people I have met, especially those of us who like to be in control of our lives. When we are in the hands of others, when we are not able to go and do what we want when we want, some of us just want to heal on our own until we are back to our normal selves. There are others who are completely different and need people around them for emotional support. If you are on your own cancer journey, be true to yourself and honest about what you need so your support people know what to do.

Marie was with Graham every step of the way. She sat by his hospital bed each day, never leaving his side for the eight weeks it took for him to heal sufficiently to be discharged.

"I'm just one of those people who puts one foot in front of the other, every day is a bonus," said Marie. "I didn't get caught up in thoughts like, 'He may be dead tomorrow' or, 'He could die' at any stage. Somebody had to be positive."

Not one to sit around feeling sorry for himself, Graham worked hard on regaining his fitness. Supported by Marie, their children and extended family, he was able to keep a positive mindset.

"Once I left hospital, it really didn't cross my mind that I was going to die. I never thought that was going to happen. I was always really positive that way."

Graham went from strength to strength, feeling good enough to return to work after six months. He continued with his regular check-ups and scans, at first every three months, then six months, then annually as there appeared to be no sign of reoccurrence.

The usual recovery time for such a major operation can be 12 months or more so I asked Graham what enabled him to bounce back and return to work so quickly. He laughed and told me it was by not following the nutritionist's advice to eat cakes and fatty foods to regain the 10 kg (22 lb) he had lost.

Graham credits his fast recovery to a combination of things: being fit before the surgery, plus a change of diet and natural therapies. He was fortunate to have been given a lot of advice by his nieces who attended health seminars in America and Germany where they had friends on the cutting edge of the latest wellness therapies. On their advice, Graham started on a healthy eating program that consisted of mostly salad. He also eliminated all meats and sugars and began drinking freshly juiced green vegetables.

In addition to his change in diet, Graham had regular colonics to boost his immune system, to alkalise his body and to improve his overall digestive system. He also had Vitamin C infusions administered intravenously to accelerate the repair and regeneration process of tissue in his body.

Everything was going well for four years until Graham's scan in 2013. He was 63 when the doctor informed him that the cancer had returned and that it was showing signs of growing again in the same area. This inevitably meant that he would have to repeat the same operation and recovery process. The diagnosis did not sit well with Graham.

"When I left hospital after the major surgery, the same doctor said, 'In 99% of the patients, we never have to do anything again', but after he told us it had returned, we did our own research and found out that generally, this thing does come back."

Graham asked for all his scans and the accompanying reports. The couple was confused at what they had been told and decided to take the reports to some other specialists to get another opinion as they were having second thoughts about repeating the procedure.

Marie compared the difference in how they felt at his first diagnosis to how they felt with the reoccurrence:

"When Graham was first diagnosed, we went in full bore, we did no research, we just did what the doctor said. You put all your trust in the doctor. We didn't know any different, they didn't give us time to think."

Now that they knew what they would be facing, Graham and Marie wanted to take the time to look at their options and make an informed choice.

Graham took his reports and asked for other opinions on his prognosis. Some specialists supported their efforts with alternative therapies, while others thought they were freaks.

The final straw came when Graham and Marie actually read through the past four years of scans and reports themselves, only to discover that the cancer had actually reappeared on the scans a whole year before they were alerted to it by their doctor!

This is Graham's one regret: that he did not check the scans and read the reports properly himself. As many people do, he trusted the doctor to interpret them and to provide the best advice.

"The tumours showed up on those scans, even the report said that cancer had returned, but he didn't say anything until a full 12 months later. If he had told me at the three-year mark, I could have started working on it a whole year earlier."

After much consideration, Graham told his doctor that he was going to try natural therapies because he did not want to go through the operation or the chemotherapy again.

Graham doubled up on all his treatments and supplements, increasing the number of colonics and Vitamin C infusions, adding enemas and a daily sauna. He also increased the supplements he takes including Vitamin B12, probiotics, enzymes, apricot kernels, dandelion tea and fermented vegetables for gut health.

While we were chatting, Graham excused himself and came back with a jar of what looked like some dirt in water. He explained, "It's clay, and it draws all of the toxins out of your body and flushes them out of your system. And the water is ionised, alkaline water."

With the number of different therapies to co-ordinate, Graham's meticulously planned treatment schedule is beyond impressive. I am in awe of the discipline he has to ensure the best possible outcome.

Marie puts it all into perspective for me by explaining the dynamics of the teamwork in their relationship:

"For Graham, everything has to run to a plan and that's how it is. I annoy Graham because I'm not organised, I've never been organised in my life. If it falls into place, it falls into place, so I've got to remind myself to be more considerate!"

Graham continued with check-ups and scans and his condition did improve a little. The tumour actually shrank, but then it did come back, encroaching on the vena cava and also the kidneys.

The doctors started putting pressure on Graham to have the second surgery and to remove one of his kidneys.

"When I decided not to have the surgery and to go in a different direction, the doctors didn't want to know me. They have virtually said I am on my own."

It is five years on from that decision, and Graham has not had a check-up or scan for two years. He feels good, so he just doesn't worry about it. Graham keeps active and helps his family with building work on their homes. He is also thinking about some renovations on his own home. Graham and Marie are making the most of every moment and keep focussed on what is most important to them—their family and grandkids.

"I feel okay for 67. I get a bit tired sometimes, but I think it goes with what I do and getting older. I just want to live my life and make the best of it all."

19

LUKE, KATIE, ELI AND HARPER

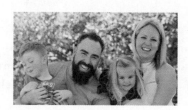

DIAGNOSIS: RETINOBLASTOMA

When I visited the Rollinsons on a Saturday afternoon, I walked into a typical family home: Mum Katie and Dad Luke are there; Eli, aged four, was excited to show me his new fluorescent orange football boots; and Harper, aged three, was watching a movie. The kids ran to the door to meet me and my good friend Julie, Luke's mother.

The ordinariness of the scene is particularly wonderful when you know the family's journey so far—they have walked through fire and emerged stronger.

Their story began 35 years ago when Julie, her husband Graham, and a then 18-month-old Luke went out for a day at the beach. As they were enjoying the sunshine, a friend commented that she noticed Luke constantly tilting his head to the side. Julie thought it was odd and the next night, Luke was restless and came in to sleep with his parents. This was very unusual behaviour for the toddler.

The next morning, Luke's eye was an angry shade of red, so Julie arranged a doctor's appointment for that afternoon. The GP immediately realised something was seriously wrong and arranged appointment with an eye specialist for that same day.

The specialist examined Luke's eye in his rooms, but as you can imagine, keeping an active child still for an examination proved difficult. The doctor decided to examine Luke under general anaesthetic and within hours, the little boy was in theatre.

It was nine o'clock at night when the specialist emerged to inform Luke's anxious parents that he was very worried about their son's eye. He asked them to take him to Camperdown Children's Hospital, now The Children's Hospital at Westmead, the next morning to see the country's leading eye specialist.

Upon their arrival at the Children's Hospital, their new specialist told Julie and Graham that Luke's right eye was full of tumour and that the only option was to remove it. To compound the situation, his left eye had two tumours, but the doctor insisted that it could be saved.

Luke's condition was diagnosed as retinoblastoma, a cancer in the retina of the eye. It is more common in children under three years of age and can affect one or both eyes. The speed with which Luke was referred on was an indication of the urgency of his case, and that same morning Luke was in theatre for surgery. Less than 48 hours after his initial doctor's appointment, Luke's right eye was gone.

"I was hysterical. One of the worst days of my life was going into recovery and seeing Luke there with this big patch over his eye, to know that he didn't have an eye there."

—Julie

Julie and Graham stayed with Luke at the hospital for two weeks. As awful as it was that Luke had his eye removed, it was a blessing that the surgery was done before it spread to the optic nerve. Doctors informed them that this may have happened within a matter of days and then the cancer would have spread throughout his whole body.

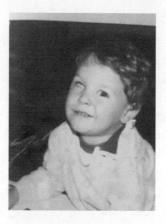

Luke after his surgery

Julie recalls the difficulty of managing their lives during this period. Back then, public awareness of cancer was virtually non-existent and the current support mechanisms that families can access were not available. Cancer was not a subject that was discussed, even with friends, so Julie and Graham handled their crisis on their own.

The logistics of fitting Luke's treatment into their lives was a challenge for the young family. They had recently moved to the Illawarra region, a two-hour drive from the Sydney hospitals equipped to treat their son. The couple were working in local jobs near their new home: Graham was the Deputy Town Planner at the newly formed Shellharbour Council and Julie was Head Art Teacher at Lake Illawarra High School. Life became a juggling act as they coped with job responsibilities and the many trips to and from hospitals in Sydney with Luke.

As luck would have it, new medical machines had arrived at the Sydney Eye Hospital shortly before Luke's diagnosis. He was one of the first patients to receive laser therapy in combination with cryotherapy. Julie and Luke would take the two-hour trip up to the hospital every six weeks for over a year. On each visit, Luke was put under general anaesthetic for treatment with these therapies. He was very young at the time, but still remembers that the environment was dull and full of old people.

Fortunately for Luke, the treatment destroyed the tumours thus eliminating the need for chemotherapy or radiation, and he maintained the sight in his left eye. Luke's check-ups started at three-month intervals and because there were no problems, they became six-monthly and then annually until he was a teenager.

Luke also returned to the Camperdown Children's Hospital regularly for chest X-rays and a Gallium scan. This continued until he was aged 12.

"Whilst I lost my right eye altogether, in some unique way, I feel lucky compared to other children who had cancer and had to undergo chemotherapy for their treatments. From meeting other people around my age who were affected by retinoblastoma, they seemed to suffer more side-effects in their ongoing lives."

— LUKE

Luke's early childhood treatment was 100% successful. I asked him what effect his cancer had on his childhood and Luke smiled as he shared a favourite anecdote. The kids at primary school would call him names for having an artificial right eye. One day, he finally got so sick of it that when a group of girls started teasing him, he took his glass eye out and began to chase them around the playground with it. Screaming and horror stories ensued, resulting in a trip with his parents to the Principal's office for a lecture about appropriate behaviour!

Apart from the regular hospital visits, Luke grew up doing everything any other child his age would do. He refused to let his affected vision hold him back in any way. Luke learnt to adapt and participated in many sports, playing football at a junior representative level.

Despite her son's success in life, Julie has always worried about what caused the cancer and why it happened.

"In one sense, I always used to blame myself that he lost his eye, because I always had really bad eyesight, and thought, 'I'd hate to have a blind kid.' It's a strange thing."

— JULIE

It was discovered that Luke's cancer could not be attributed to anything that Julie had eaten or done during pregnancy; it was just bad luck, and no one could have predicted its occurrence. When both Julie and Graham were tested, neither of them had the cancer RB1 gene. Sydney University conducted a study into retinoblastoma as it was a rare form of cancer. They concluded that it was caused by the combination of Graham and Julie's genes creating a rogue cell in Luke.

Now 36 years old, Luke maintains good vision in his left eye and has remained cancer-free since those early childhood days. The only things that bother him today are minor: due to his glass eye, sometimes his line of sight may be a little off when he is talking to people, and when driving he may need to turn his head a little more than the average person to see a blind spot.

Luke married the beautiful Katie and the young couple was excited to have their first child, Eli. He was four months old when Katie noticed that Eli's left pupil appeared white in a flash photograph. Known as cat's eye reflex or leukocoria, this unusual whiteness is one of the tell-tale signs of cancer in the retina.

Upon investigation, Eli was found to have a small tumour on the outer edge of his left eye, the exact same cancer that Luke had dealt with over three decades earlier. The new parents were absolutely gutted.

Prior to having children, both Luke and Katie were aware that there was a possibility that Luke's childhood retinoblastoma could be genetically passed onto their children. But getting access to the right information and tangible advice on these possibilities was something never offered or made available to them.

Luke's one regret is that prior to having children, he did not definitively know that his childhood retinoblastoma could be genetically passed on to his children.

"To be honest, we were a little ignorant of the chances of me passing on the retinoblastoma gene to our kids. We knew there was a slight chance, given my history, but we weren't sure if my cancer was the random kind or the genetic kind."

— Luke

Eli underwent both laser therapy and cryotherapy treatment, similar to his father, at Westmead Children's Hospital. Due to the fact that the tumour was discovered earlier, the treatment eradicated the abnormal cells and Eli has sight in both eyes. Like his father, Eli has avoided the harshness of chemotherapy and radiotherapy to date.

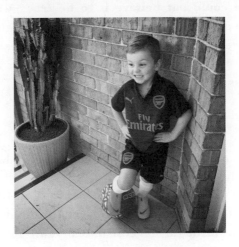

Eli in his football boots

In dealing with the appropriate specialists at Westmead Children's Hospital for Eli, it became obvious that genetic testing should be conducted to identify the commonality between father and son. The results confirmed that both Luke and Eli carry a mutation of the RB1 gene. This information immediately sparked questions of how it would affect any future children. Luke and Katie were informed there was a 50% chance that the gene would be passed on and a 50% chance that the carrier would then develop the eye cancer.

In preparing for their second child, this information was not reassuring so they sought advice from various geneticists and specialists on available approaches. The option of conceiving with IVF was a possibility, as the gene could be isolated and removed to avoid any chance of the cancer being passed. But at the time, this was understood to be extremely expensive and unfeasible for the couple, and it would also be quite invasive for Katie. Instead, they worked with doctors at both Westmead Children's Hospital and Wollongong Hospital to prepare a plan for their next child involving in utero genetic testing.

When Katie discovered she was pregnant, the plan went into motion. At 19 weeks into her pregnancy, Katie had an amniocentesis to find out if her baby carried the gene. The test results were positive; the baby girl she carried could also be born with the same cancer.

"Whilst we could not believe it to be true—what are the chances we could have two kids with cancer, right? We put a plan in place with our Wollongong and Westmead doctors to deliver our baby early and check her eyes for tumours as soon as possible."

— LUKE

No words could describe the emotions that Katie and Luke experienced in the following 18 weeks.

"It's the not knowing and the uncertainty that is the hard thing to go through. It consumes you. You just want someone to tell you it's going to be okay, but at the end of the day, it doesn't always happen."

— LUKE

Knowing how aggressive the cancer could be, their beautiful little girl Harper was delivered at 36 weeks.

Unlike other families that prepare to take their precious new baby home only a few days after birth, Luke and Katie faced the dread of knowing that their child's birth could be the beginning of a new challenge.

Eight days after her birth, doctors found a large tumour behind Harper's right eye. Upon consultation with the medical team at Westmead, Luke and Katie were told that Harper needed chemotherapy immediately. When children and babies have chemotherapy, the side-effects can be very serious, including hearing loss and temporary or permanent damage to vital organs.

"To say Katie and I were devastated was an understatement. Being a parent, all you want for your kids is for them to be healthy, and not knowing what would come of such treatment for our fragile, tiny, newborn baby girl, was just heartbreaking for us. She was just so small and so little. It was just no way for someone to be welcomed into this world. I remember thinking, 'How could life be so cruel for something so innocent?' But it was what it was, and we had no choice but to face this head on and do our best to be there for our little girl."

— LUKE

Harper was just 12 days old when she started treatment. At the time, she was the second-youngest baby to start chemotherapy at Westmead Children's Hospital. Her treatment involved six rounds of chemotherapy spread over six months, incorporating long stays and visits at Westmead which was a two-hour drive from their home.

She also needed numerous visits and stays at Wollongong Hospital, closer to home. During this period, Harper and her family made more than 40 single-day trips to these hospitals for blood transfusions, testing and sickness.

"The first two rounds of chemotherapy were the most difficult, which was a bit of an unknown for the doctors as she fell well below her birth weight, being so small and young."

— KATIE

Katie recalls the time when Harper was admitted to Wollongong Hospital and tube-fed until she gained some weight. Chemotherapy treatments continued until Harper was six-months old, with treatment, monitoring and general health issues being faced every round. Luckily for Harper, the treatment was medically deemed a success, as the tumour was gone.

I asked Luke and Katie how these multiple crises impacted their daily life. They both expressed gratitude for their generous support network. Both Luke and Katie held responsible jobs with the same firm, MMJ Wollongong, Luke as Director of Town Planning and Katie as National Marketing Manager. They felt blessed that they were given the time and space to focus on their family with the company's partners taking care of things during their absence.

Luke explains that period in their lives as being as if someone had pushed the 'pause' button on their regular life. He recalls spending night after night with Katie next to Harper's bed in hospital, and their accommodating family members caring for Eli and making the four-hour round trip up to the hospital and back home again so that the family could all be together.

During these long periods in hospital, both Luke and Katie got to know other families in similar situations. They noticed that most children only had one parent at the hospital as the other had to go to work. How difficult it must be as a parent to go to work when all you would want is to be at your child's bedside.

The family was supported by loved ones, friends and even the kindness of strangers. Katie was a member of an expectant mothers Facebook group and the group's organiser, Cassie Fersterer, was so moved by Katie's story that she set up a GoFundMe page. The story attracted national media attention and featured on the Today Show, with the campaign raising over $80,000. Luke expressed his heartfelt gratitude on his Facebook page:

"Thank you to the Today Show for sharing our story and to Cassie Fersterer for everything she has done. Also, can't thank everyone enough for supporting our little family during this time. Words can't explain how much we appreciate it!"

— Luke

It was not the money per se, but what it was able to do for them. When your life is totally disrupted, the basic chores of life still need to get done and, in a crisis situation, these are not top of mind. With the funds raised, Cassie arranged for a meal delivery service so that Luke and Katie could focus all their energy on the wellbeing of their children. The funds raised also enabled the purchase of an air-conditioning purification system for Harper's room.

In addition, the family received assistance from various not-for-profit organisations such as Camp Quality and Redkite. Camp Quality arranged for a cleaner to attend to Luke and Katie's home for a six-week period whilst they both ran back and forth from hospital. Redkite would often supply the couple with fuel and food vouchers.

"For us, these organisations provided amazing support services, and still do to date. It's the little things that you just never forget."

— LUKE

Camp Quality is an amazing organisation and one of the few that focusses on providing emotional support. Their purpose, to build optimism and resilience for kids and their families who are impacted by cancer, is fulfilled in many practical ways. Along with arranging cleaning services, Camp Quality invited the Rollinsons on a trip to Perisher, one of Australia's most popular holiday destinations. It was a wonderful chance for them to meet other families experiencing the same challenges and to understand that they were not going through the journey alone. Camp Quality arranged everything including qualified caregivers, to allow parents to have a break and a chance to recoup their energy.

Luke and Katie acknowledge their appreciation of these organisations by giving their time and effort to fundraising. In the last two years, Luke has participated in the 12-hour cycle ride and raised close to $50,000 for the Children's Cancer Institute (CCI).

The family has been an ambassador for the Cancer Council's Relay for Life in Wollongong and has also been invited to speak at various charity events for both Camp Quality and CCI. Luke is, to this day, very involved with Camp Quality and recently spoke at a Federal Government breakfast briefing in support of this organisation.

"For us, it is important to tell our story and help those organisations that we believe in or have helped us personally. If we can use our story to help other families going through childhood cancer treatment or even prevent it altogether, then why wouldn't we. It's the least we could do."

— LUKE

Harper is now three years old. The chemotherapy was successful, but it did cause severe hearing loss as an unfortunate side-effect. She started using hearing aids at age two, which provided some benefit in terms of volume. They did, however, lack the clarity she needed to improve her speech. This caused Harper's development to fall behind other children her age.

It was suggested to Luke and Katie that they consider cochlear implants as a solution. As the procedure is irreversible, making the decision for Harper at such a young age was quite a difficult one.

After much consideration, and strong recommendations from various specialists, they decided to go ahead with the five-hour surgery and just before Christmas 2017, her implants were activated. Harper's reaction was priceless!

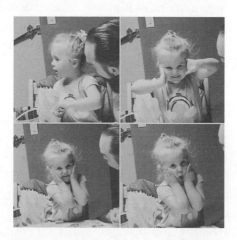

Harper reacting to her new cochlear implants!

Cancer is a journey and, for this family, it continues with regular check-ups. A hospital visit in the life of the Rollinsons involves a 5.30am start and a day of fasting that Luke and Katie do with the kids. It usually ends up being a 12-hour day, with a lot of waiting to see doctors before and after testing under general anaesthetic. It is always challenging to keep two active kids calm and amused while they are extremely hungry!

The hardest part is waiting for the results and worrying about the outcome. It is always such a relief to get the 'all clear'. These check-ups will continue to be a part of their lives and, though physically and mentally draining, the Rollinsons attend them with grateful hearts and a positive attitude.

"Every time our minds wandered to the what ifs and the worst-case scenarios, I remembered Dad's advice: 'Try not to think too far ahead. Don't worry about what you don't know or what could happen. Just deal with the facts that you do know.'"

— LUKE

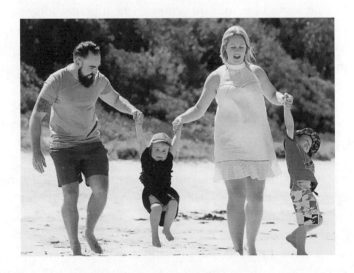

20

MARK

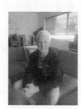

Diagnosis: Bladder Cancer

Mark and his wife Jo live in a beautiful part of Australia located two hours south of Sydney and just a street back from the beach. The day I met Mark he invited me into their home which he proudly tells me he built. The house is beautifully designed, with spectacular views over the water. A builder for all of his working life, Mark is now retired. He looks amazingly fit and I would never guess that he had major surgery just a year ago.

The first symptom that alerted Mark to his illness occurred around the middle of 2016, when he was 61 years old. He noticed that there was blood in his urine and with a trip booked to go overseas two days later, he thought he should get it checked out before he left.

He managed to arrange an appointment with his GP and after explaining the problem, the doctor performed a litmus test on his urine and suspected a bladder infection. She prescribed antibiotics and assured Mark he was fine to travel and that it would probably clear up within a few days. Relieved that it would not interfere with their plans, Mark started taking the medication and embarked on the trip to the 2016 Rio Olympics as intended.

Following the Olympics, the couple had arranged a stopover in Las Vegas. Mark's problem was getting worse to the point where he sought medical help while he was in the 'City of Lights'. The physician advised him to go to a specialist as soon as he arrived home.

If there was one piece of luck for Mark, it was that his wife's cousin was the medical receptionist for a respected urologist. She was able to book him in for an appointment fairly quickly and at his first consultation, the specialist told him to throw away the antibiotics and promptly sent him off to have an ultrasound and a CT scan.

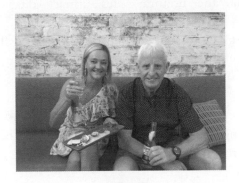

Jo and Mark

The test results showed a 50 mm (2 in) tumour in Mark's bladder. It was an aggressive form of cancer and surgery was booked for the following week. The doctor explained that he would be cutting it out, adding that it was one of the better places to have cancer because the thickness of the bladder wall would allow him to go deep and scrape out all the cancer cells.

At this point, Mark felt he was in good hands, trusting that the tumour would be successfully removed, that he would make a fast recovery and quickly get back to his normal life. It did not turn out that way. This initial surgery became the first step in a much more challenging journey than expected.

Despite the surgeon's best efforts, he was not absolutely sure that he had removed all the cancerous cells in Mark's bladder. He was concerned that he had needed to cut so deeply that he almost went through the outside wall of Mark's bladder. To give his patient the best prognosis, the doctor advised that further treatment would be required, and that Mark would need to choose from two options.

The first option was to have chemotherapy and radiotherapy, and statistics showed that this treatment offered an average of an additional 10 years of life.

The other option was a far more radical procedure and involved the complete removal of Mark's existing bladder and the construction of a new bladder, known as a neobladder. It is made by taking a piece of intestine (bowel) which is the shape of a tube, opening it lengthways, shaping it into a bladder and then stitching it together. It is then positioned where the bladder was previously situated and attached to the ureters and the urethra. This urinary diversion allows the preservation of as much normal function as possible.

Due to Mark's fitness, age and healthy Body Mass Index (BMI), his specialist recommended the neo bladder as a better option, because statistics suggest an additional 30 quality years of life as a result of this procedure.

Mark had complete faith in his medical team and the option of a long and healthy life made the decision easy for him. He had no interest in researching further information or dwelling on the choice for days on end.

"He said I could go home and look it up on Dr Google, but I never did. I didn't even read the pages about what can go wrong. All I was worried about was that when something went wrong, he could fix it."

Jo was the one who read the information and did the research. Her concern was born out of past experience, as her father died of bladder cancer. Now that it was happening to her husband, she wanted to make sure they were making the right choices.

The doctor was quite confident that the neobladder would give him the best chance at a cancer-free life. Mark agreed, and his surgery took place in November 2016.

It was much worse than Mark had expected. After the 10-hour surgery, he emerged with drains to bags from his kidneys and abdomen. He had a catheter in his new bladder, a port in his chest and an IV line to administer medication and nutrition.

"I lost 15.5 kg (34 lb), I just didn't feel like eating. They tried to give me tablets and I just spewed everything up."

There was a further complication that occurred shortly after he was released from ICU to a general ward. The bottom of his heart was beating extremely fast, while the top section was beating normally. A whole group of specialists appeared at the end of his bed and Mark recalls with amusement how they were arguing about what to do with him and who among them was responsible for doing it. He had never experienced any previous issues with his heart, and tests showed that his veins were exceptionally clear for a man his age. They ended up giving him some medication which he is still on today.

It was a horrendous experience for Mark. Recovery from such serious surgery is a challenge not just physically, but mentally. Not being in control of his own basic needs destroyed his sense of dignity.

"I started to get the shits and I just wanted to end it. I was tired. I hardly slept. I couldn't see myself coming good. I thought, 'No one can live like this.'"

Mark did not want to see any visitors because he was too tired to speak more than a few words. Thankfully, he had the love and support of Jo and their three adult children. Jo was at the hospital every day during his month-long stay and his son cut short a holiday in New Zealand to come home and support his father.

"My family put in an incredible effort. If it wasn't for my family, I don't know, I would probably...I don't know what. You need that support. They've all been very good."

Mark was released from hospital with one of the drains and bags still connected to his neobladder. This was due to an inherent issue with constructing a bladder from intestinal material. A normal function of the intestine is to produce mucus, a filmy substance that assists in excreting waste from the intestines. It is also a muscle that continuously works to push food through the system. These two factors still occur when the tissue is constructed into a bladder and if not continuously flushed, the neobladder can become blocked with the mucus.

"I still had the bag two months later because I think they feel more at ease that it's not going to block because when that is removed, you're on your own."

Once Mark did have the bag removed, the next battle was learning how to function with the changes to his body. His new bladder could only hold around 400 ml (13.5 oz), so that meant that he needed to empty it regularly. He also needed to drink water frequently to keep flushing the mucus through his new bladder and most importantly, he had to work out what signal his body was now giving when he needed to go to the toilet—the previous trigger mechanism went with his original bladder.

It was a tricky process to learn. Mark has mastered it now, describing it as a certain pain in his stomach that now indicates he needs to empty his bladder. The most difficult time is sleeping as he no longer has the trigger to wake up if he needs to go to the toilet in the middle of the night, though he has solved this by setting an alarm to wake up and go to the bathroom around 1am.

He has been a good steward of his neobladder, in part due to his chat with a man who underwent the same cystectomy and bladder reconstruction at the age of 35. Apparently, this man had not heeded medical advice and his neobladder had blocked three times. On the third occasion he was drunk, went to sleep and woke up when it burst. That man has had to go through the entire reconstruction procedure again, a hard lesson to learn.

Around three months after surgery, just when he was starting to feel better, Mark started chemotherapy. He had infusions every Monday and Wednesday for two consecutive weeks, then one week off. This cycle continued for a six-month period.

"I think the chemo was worse than the surgery. I used to have good veins, the best one in my arm used to pop out, but now they have all gone into hiding because they don't want any more chemo going in."

Mark has also had issues with blood clots in his legs, taking blood thinners and administering himself with daily anticoagulant injections to prevent them. He believes it is a consequence of the chemotherapy and it is an ongoing problem. Despite these complications, it is incredible how quickly he has recovered. He has put 10 kg (22 lb) back on and feels much better for it.

"Exercise has helped my recovery unbelievably. Fitness and being healthy has always been a part of my life and I think that made the difference. I think it comes down to doing something. I said to myself, 'You can just sit on the lounge all day long if you want, but you've just got to get out there and do it.'"

Today Mark is moving forward and improving in leaps and bounds. He cycles and walks a total of 20 km (12 mi) every day. Jo is equally active and still competes in iron woman events at age 62. The couple love the beach and Mark is excited to be back into surfing and doing all the things he loves with his friends and family.

"We're not here long and when you've had cancer and you look at your age you think, 'I better do something about this.' I'm just cramming as much as I can in. I'm going to jam everything I can in. I go fishing with my mates. I play with my grandkids. Before I thought, 'I won't worry about it, I'll wait another week.' Now I just go."

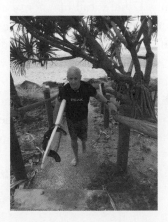

21

LINDA

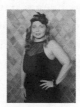

DIAGNOSIS: ANAL CANCER

Linda is a woman of substance who has battled unbelievable odds and overcome challenges that would have defeated others. Linda accurately describes herself as an autoimmune disease warrior and cancer survivor; nothing will stop her from thriving!

Linda is 39 years old and her story begins 19 years ago when she was aged 20. Set on a career path devoted to helping others in the community services sector, she was a hard worker with a close circle of good friends and family. Usually full of energy and enthusiasm, Linda started experiencing extreme fatigue and digestive issues. She had severe abdominal pain and at one point, her total body weight dropped to just 32 kg (70 lb).

Seeking medical help, Linda was admitted to her local hospital in Wollongong. The medical staff conducted a thorough range of tests and could not find a diagnosis. What made Linda's case more mysterious was that the symptoms would come and go.

"I was in hospital for six weeks. They told me I was crazy

or depressed. I said, 'I'm not depressed. There's something wrong with me.'"

The doctors finally diagnosed Linda with Crohn's disease a few days before she was released from hospital. Her medical team recommended surgery to remove her colon, but one doctor felt she was too young for such a radical solution. He sent Linda to a variety of specialists in Sydney including gastroenterologists and surgeons. No one could offer an alternative therapy until she was finally referred to a specialist in Royal Prince Alfred Hospital (RPA) in Sydney. This doctor was the leading specialist in Crohn's disease and he referred her to a colorectal surgeon. Through the collaboration of these two doctors, Linda was relieved to finally receive the news that she would not require a permanent stoma.

There is no cure for Crohn's disease and the exact cause is unknown, though factors of heredity and a malfunctioning immune system are thought to play a role. The disease can be controlled by medication, but in Linda's case, it had reached the stage of requiring surgical intervention.

The colorectal surgeon suggested a surgery called a j-pouch reconstruction procedure where the rectum is removed, then the bowel is reconnected to the anal canal. The surgery was successful and, though her Crohn's disease was not cured, Linda was able to control some of the symptoms with immune-suppressants and anti-inflammatories.

The most difficult part of the process was dealing with her self-esteem and body image.

"I had to have a colostomy bag for a while and it was difficult, being that young. The worst thing was body image because you're worried about getting boyfriends at that age. Even if someone approached me, I would be like, get away, you don't want to deal with me."

Linda attributes the support of her family, especially her mother, and her close friends for helping her through this stage of her life.

Over the years, as is typical with Crohn's disease, symptoms would flare up, then at other times, they would be less severe. Linda tried many different medications to control it, including a drug called Humira which gave her medically induced lupus, an extremely rare side effect.

"If the textbook says a person will experience this, and only one in a thousand people will experience it, that will be me."

Linda kept searching for answers and found a naturopath who was able to help her.

"When I went back to the specialist, I didn't actually tell him about the naturopath because sometimes they're a little bit funny about it. He looked at my scan and my colonoscopy and said, 'Hmmm. Whatever you're doing, keep doing it!' And I said, 'I will!'"

Around 15 years after her j-pouch surgery, Linda had become a committed workaholic. Even when she developed serious symptoms including swollen legs, passing excessive urine and frequent vomiting, she ignored it all thinking that her ailments were related to Crohn's disease. Most people would have rushed to the doctor, but Linda continued going to work as usual.

"I tried to fight against it for ages. I needed to go to work, I needed money to pay the bills and my body just shut down. It decided it was not doing that anymore."

Fortunately, Linda had an appointment with her GP to pick up a prescription for some antibiotics. He took one look at her swollen legs and sent her for a scan. The radiology staff told her to go straight back to her GP, but Linda returned to work instead. When she did not arrive, the GP called her wondering why she hadn't come to see him. When she finally got to the GP, he sent her away with instructions to drop everything and get to a hospital. Linda responded, "Do I really have to go now?"

She finally agreed and drove herself to RPA Hospital. The moment Linda walked into emergency she was swamped by six doctors who told her that total kidney failure was imminent because she was walking around with only 5% function.

Linda was put on kidney dialysis immediately. This is something that she continues to do today, three days a week for five hours on each of those days. Linda muses that it is the equivalent of a part time job.

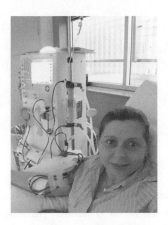

Linda having her dialysis treatment

Prior to her kidney failure, Linda's Crohn's disease symptoms had settled down, but a few months into dialysis, some issues arose that caused her to have emergency surgery. Linda ended up with a stoma again and was getting discharge and frequent infections. When she informed her surgeon, he dismissed her concerns, advising that it would subside. Despite complaining about the same problem several times over the following years, she was not treated and Linda wonders if that contributed to her cancer diagnosis.

If this wasn't enough to deal with, Linda's apartment building caught on fire due to an electrical fault. The roof collapsed and the entire building came down. She lost everything and though it was devastating at the time, it turned out to be a blessing in disguise.

Linda's medical team began the workup for a kidney transplant. Aged just 37, she was a good candidate, but they were concerned about her Crohn's disease issues and her ongoing fistula. Linda went back to her specialist at the RPA Hospital and he arranged for her to have several tests including scans and a biopsy. The biopsy came back positive with cancer (squamous-cell carcinoma) in the anal canal.

"I was in shock, I think, because I just went quiet. I was thinking to myself, 'I'm calm.' It was like I was waiting for a reaction to happen, but nothing was happening. It was a bit of a non-event."

Her reaction was so low-key that Linda remembers the doctor saying, "You know this is serious? If you don't do something you're going to die." Linda's Mum accompanied her to all her appointments and she too was quiet, stunned at what the doctor was saying. The pair left the doctor's office with a referral to an oncologist who arranged a regime of chemotherapy and radiation treatment.

I asked Linda if the full impact of her diagnosis affected her emotionally at any stage.

"The hardest thing was telling my brother because he was overseas at the time. I'd been putting little posts on Facebook, but I didn't want him to see it there, I needed to tell him myself. He happened to call home that day because he remembered I was getting my biopsy results and I had to tell him."

Linda was preparing to start radiation when the specialists called her back to discuss a surgical intervention. Once they had reviewed her scans again, Linda's medical team felt that the radiation would flare up her Crohn's disease. Along with her non-functioning kidneys, her bladder was not working, and her previous diagnosis of high-grade VIN and CIN3, combined with the long-term use of immune suppressants, put Linda at high risk of developing cervical cancer.

The recommended course of action was for Linda to have a Total Pelvic Exenteration: the removal of her bladder, bowel, ovaries, womb, cervix, vagina and rectum.

The surgical procedure took 15 hours: 11 hours for the removal of organs, then four hours for the plastic surgeon to do his work. The procedure went well for Linda; the surgeon managed to remove the whole tumour within the margins and there was nothing in the lymph nodes, so she did not need to have any chemotherapy or radiation. Linda's only complication was with the plastic surgery, which required a further operation at a later stage.

Linda had a week in ICU before transferring to the ward where she spent around four weeks, starting on a fluid diet plus intravenous nutrition. The first few days were very painful with Linda unable to lie on her back or her front. She could not sit for many weeks and had to either stand or lie on her side. Then came the challenge of getting up and walking without splitting her stitches. Linda worked with a physiotherapist, starting with little shuffle steps and gradually improving day by day.

Upon her discharge from hospital, Linda's Mum took care of her.

"My Mum was really good. Behind my back she probably had a cry, but in front of me she was always really strong and positive, saying, 'We're going to do this. It's going to be alright.'"

Living with her family gave Linda the time to heal without financial pressure. She had stopped working when her kidneys failed so moving in with her Mum after the fire burned down her apartment was a godsend. Another thing Linda is thankful for is having private health insurance from a young age. This paid for all her medical expenses, gave her the ability to choose her own doctors, and to be treated as a private patient.

Her extended Italian family and close friends have supported Linda throughout her journey. When she thought she would require chemotherapy and radiation, her best friend, who lived close to the hospital, offered to take care of her and opened up her home to Linda.

"I had good people around me all the time, people that would lift me up. Even if I had a down day, they would always try and help me, to pick me up."

Today Linda is 18 months on from that surgery and looks really well. She is cancer-free, and has her sights set on the five-year mark as that will allow her to become eligible for a kidney transplant. I asked her what she has done to make such an excellent recovery.

"At first, I kind of buried my head in the sand. I just let the doctors do what they wanted to do. Then I started to do some research afterwards."

Linda searched for ways to speed up her recovery and to deal with the ongoing Crohn's disease symptoms. From the information she found, Linda changed her diet and began to eat wholefoods, choosing organic where possible. One of the biggest battles she has is maintaining weight and consuming the high amount of protein she needs. Linda credits Isagenix shakes as key in helping her digest protein in a liquid form so that she can metabolise the nutrients and keep at a healthy weight.

Other therapies Linda has explored include essential oils, and she swears by frankincense, an anti-inflammatory oil that she finds works particularly well. Linda has also engaged in the Complementary Therapy and Supportive Care Unit at the Chris O'Brien Lifehouse where cancer patients can access yoga, mindfulness meditation, reflexology, qi gong, physiotherapy and more.

Despite everything she has been through, it is Linda's positive attitude that is exceptional. She does not complain about her situation, nor does she describe any experience as difficult or too hard. She has accepted what is and gets on with what she wants to do. How does she do it?

"I always have a goal, I guess. Something to look forward to. Instead of worrying about the past, I think about the future, about getting there and what I need to do to get there."

Linda's personal journey of discovery has influenced her decision to study food and nutrition and her goal is to become qualified to share that knowledge with others. She is currently in the process of attaining her Bachelor of Food and Nutrition through La Trobe University.

"I was a workaholic. When I was having those problems, I thought, 'I've got to go to work. I have to do this. I have to do that.' Don't worry about work. Listen to what your body is telling you. If it's telling you there's something wrong, just do what you need to do to heal it."

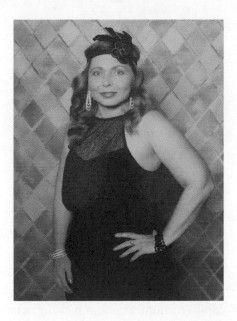

22

ADAM

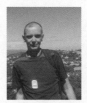

Diagnosis: Tongue Cancer

It is hard to imagine the devastation Adam felt when he first discovered he had tongue cancer. Any cancer diagnosis is shocking, but for someone who is a good communicator, it was overwhelming to have his cancer affect the very organ that gives us speech.

Adam chose a customer service career, starting his working life as a retail bookshop manager, specialising in commercial and residential architecture and building. He loved his job: interacting with clients, building relationships and sourcing the right books for them. Adam became an accomplished book buyer, attending the largest book fair in the world held at Frankfurt, Germany, as well as American book fairs in Los Angeles and New York.

His cancer journey began two years after he returned to his native country of New Zealand. Aged 41, Adam had several weeks of unexplained tooth pain that led to a biopsy, and subsequently, to a diagnosis of squamous cell carcinoma at the base of his tongue.

Adam was terrified. He recalls bursting into tears and asking the specialist how long he had to live. His doctor assured him, "If you are going to get tongue cancer, this is the one you want," because it can be treated with a combination of chemotherapy and aggressive radiation.

There is no tongue cancer that anyone wants, and Adam found himself trying to process the implications of his diagnosis, while preparing to face the treatment to come.

"When you are told you have cancer, life goes on hold and the end of your life suddenly has a time frame. A fog descends. It's like living, but not living."

Due to the position of Adam's cancer, he was sent to have a mask made to fit the contours of his face. He watched as they heated up a flat piece of plastic mesh to mould over his face and shoulders. Once in place, they covered the plastic with cold towels to instantly cool and harden the plastic. The resulting mask was fitted with a surrounding piece that has clips attached and these were used to fasten Adam onto the radiation table so that he would not move during the treatment.

In addition to the mask, Adam underwent a tracheotomy prior to radiation treatment. This surgery was performed to ensure that if Adam's tongue became too swollen during treatment, the incision directly into his windpipe would ensure he could breathe.

Radiation therapy began just 10 days after his diagnosis. It was the equivalent of a full-time job: Adam attended the Oncology department at Auckland Hospital five days a week for six weeks. Each treatment involved him lying down on the table, then having the mask clipped into place over his face to keep his head restrained and perfectly still while the radiation machine burned into him for 25 minutes.

The process took some getting used to—Adam's main concern was drowning in his own phlegm while locked into position. Over the six-week period, he had to push the button for assistance twice so that he could sit up and cough up the phlegm.

On the third week of treatment, evidence of radiation damage started to appear. Adam's neck appeared sunburnt and this became multiple sores and blisters. Five different types of sores developed on his neck, each requiring different types of ointment and bandages.

The radiation also affected his mouth, with ulcers and severe gum pain. Adam was given morphine to deal with the pain, but once his dosage reached 300 mg, his medical team tried other pain medications administered orally and through pumps. The pain became so overwhelming that Adam was admitted to hospital periodically so that the pain management team could monitor him.

Pain medication, particularly morphine, created its own set of problems and Adam found himself switching between pills for constipation and pills for diarrhoea. And then there were the pills to deal with the side-effects of other medications he was taking including pills to protect his stomach lining from all the of the other pills! At one point, Adam was taking 76 pills a day and required a spreadsheet to keep track of them all.

Chemotherapy made Adam so weak that, even walking across the room required great effort. He could not swallow food during his treatment and was fitted with a Percutaneous Endoscopic Gastrostomy (P.E.G.) feeding tube to keep up his nutrition levels during and after treatment. At 1.89 m (6 ft 2 in) tall, and 76 kg (168 lb) before treatment, Adam shrank to just 48 kg (106 lb) after treatment.

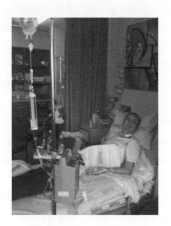

Adam during treatment

The physical and emotional trauma of Adam's treatment is beyond what most of us can imagine. He had to trust his doctors and believe in what they were doing. With no other frame of reference, Adam wondered, "Will I survive or will cancer win?"

A key component in helping Adam to endure these months of arduous treatment was the support team he had around him.

Throughout his journey Adam's main carer was his partner Mark. The two had only met eight months prior to Adam's diagnosis, and upon realising what lay ahead, Adam offered Mark the option of ending their relationship. Mark did not consider it for a moment and he has stood by Adam every step of the way. At the time of Adam's diagnosis, Mark was studying nursing and his expertise and love kept Adam going during the toughest times.

Adam's mother was supportive in her own way. She preferred not to visit Adam in hospital but would often spend time with him at home. To keep his mind occupied during recovery and recuperation, Adam began a hobby building LEGO Star Wars sets, and his mother would often build LEGO with him. It became a wonderful mother and son bonding experience.

As far as friends were concerned, Adam found that there were two distinct reactions to his situation: his best friends in Australia kept in touch and were supportive through Facebook, while the few New Zealand friends he had made "ran for the hills." To Adam it was a clear indication of the strength (or otherwise) of their friendships.

One person who became an integral part of Adam's recovery was a District Nurse who visited Adam at home during treatment. She was the only medical person who gave Adam the facts about what he was about to go through and now they are best friends. She has had her own cancer journey and Adam appreciates that she is tough in her honest, genuine and caring way. Adam nominated her for a prestigious Auckland District Health Board award which she received.

Adam's other companions were of the canine variety. Mark's dog, Mac, was there for part of the journey, but it was Lucky Star, Adam's gorgeous and fabulous miniature poodle, who became his best friend and a pivotal part of his recovery.

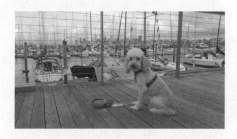

Lucky Star

Even when Adam did not feel like getting out of bed, the need to walk Lucky Star forced him to make the effort. At first, they walked to the letterbox, and then a little bit further each day. Now they bike ride 5 km (3 mi) together every day.

Many months after his treatment had finished, Adam went back to the specialist for his check-up. Adam did his best to keep positive and refused to allow negative thoughts to fill his mind. His feeling of apprehension and combination of fear and hope could be tentatively compared to other pivotal life-changing events we experience in our lives: students waiting for entrance acceptances that will determine their life careers; marriage proposals; the birth of a healthy child. In this case, the burning question for Adam was: will I be cancer free?

The camera was inserted into Adam's throat to take a look around. He was totally on edge until the surgeon confirmed that there were no signs of the tumour.

"I may be cancer free, but I have realised that I will be dealing with the side-effects for the rest of my life."

I am staggered by the effects that Adam's treatment has had on totally unrelated areas of his physical health. His chemotherapy regime caused massive hearing loss and now Adam wears hearing aids.

"I remember coming home with my new ears and crying when I heard the birds sing. It was such a wonderful sound to hear again."

The radiation treatment caused damage to Adam's tongue, throat, neck and teeth, leaving him with the inability to make saliva or to swallow. Saliva is a one of those bodily functions that is easy to take for granted, yet it is vital to help us chew and swallow, to lubricate the inside of the mouth, to create smoother speech, to dissolve food and allow the tongue to taste food.

Despite these difficulties, Adam was keen to have his P.E.G. removed completely within 12 months, rather than having it replaced with a new one. He set a goal to transfer to manual mouth feeding within that timeframe, but making this happen took a lot of effort, determination and therapy for Adam to learn how to function and thrive in his post treatment condition.

As saliva assists in neutralising the acids that break down tooth enamel, a lack of this important function meant that dental care became a major issue. To help remedy and improve his oral health and specifically, blood flow to the jaw area, Adam spent two and a half hours a day for six weeks in a Hyperbaric Oxygen Chamber at the Auckland Naval Base. He also had to relearn how to swallow, otherwise eating would be impossible. Adam worked with a speech therapist to regain this function, and he actually achieved his goal within 11 months and had his P.E.G. removed.

The next challenge became one of increasing and maintaining weight without tube feeding. It became a daily struggle as his weight wavered between 49 kg (108 lb) and 51.5 kg (114 lb).

Five years on, he has had the P.E.G. reinstalled, but the good news is that Adam's weight is up to 72 kg (159 lb) and he is feeling much more like his old self. His ribs do not show like they did, his face has filled out and his energy levels are much improved. Adam admits that he probably should not have been in such a hurry to remove the P.E.G. —hindsight is a wonderful thing!

Adam has also struggled with depression, a common development after trauma. He admits it has been a huge struggle since his cancer journey began and is very aware of the constant need to improve his mental health. I particularly love Adam's one-word mantra: engage.

With this in mind, Adam searched for a support group. He was surprised that there did not seem to be any online groups showing up on his internet searches, and he eventually contacted the Cancer Society of NZ who informed him of a small group that met on a monthly basis in Auckland. He attended their last meeting of 2016.

"It was fantastic to meet some people who understand the huge, life-changing effects of having radiation through your head and neck."

That meeting had only eight people in attendance, but it made a tremendous difference to Adam, knowing he now had contact with others who had endured the same experiences. Realising that other head and neck cancer survivors, like himself, may be finding it difficult to connect to a group, Adam offered to work with the committee to create the Head and Neck Survivors Network NZ Facebook Group and today there are 314 members.

He is involved with all the group's activities, including monthly meetings, connecting with members and advising on internet and technology matters. Adam reviews phone apps such as Cancer Aid, an app created to help cancer patients manage and improve their journeys. He is also part of the Auckland District Health Board Working Group for restructuring the way that head and neck cancer patients are treated from the beginning to the end of their treatment as well as what happens in the post treatment phase.

Adam's journey continues as he steadily builds up his fitness and improves his mental health. He is determined to engage with life instead of watching it pass him by. I have so much respect for his work with the health system and the support group to improve the experience of all cancer patients.

"Cancer is an emotional roller coaster ride. Do what all the health professionals tell you to do. Keep an open mind. Connect with others who have the same cancer. Set up a support team. Get a dog to keep you active. Engage with your health team, make decisions with them. Research your cancer, find out everything you can and use the knowledge of those who have led the way before you. Rest when you have to, get active again after treatment, get help with depression and never, never be afraid to ask for help."

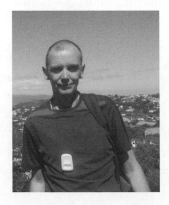

23

THE WOLLONGONG YWCA ENCORE GROUP

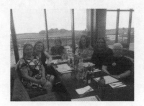

DIAGNOSIS: BREAST CANCER

This beautiful group of ladies met through YWCA Encore, an exercise program designed specifically for women who have experienced breast cancer. Apart from the health benefits they enjoy from the program, it is the friendships and connection with others who have travelled the same journey that is the true gift cherished by each of them.

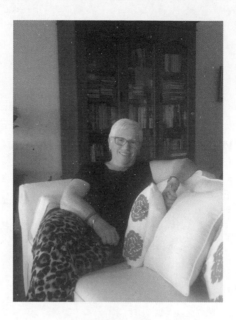

ANNETTE

A vibrant and energetic 68-year-old, Annette led an exciting life in the banking industry through which she met the love of her life, Terry, an American Naval Officer. She enjoyed most of the 1980s living in the US before returning to Australia to continue her career.

Annette faced the long-term illness of loved ones prior to her own journey and she believes that this shaped her attitude as a patient. As a daughter, she watched her mother care for her father for over six years and, as a wife, she cared for her husband, a strong man who thought he could beat his illness and worked right up until the day he passed.

When Annette was diagnosed with Grade 3 Breast Cancer at the age of 62, there was no indication of a problem. She had simply attended her routine mammogram, something she had done every two years since she was 50.

"There was no lump, no visible signs, so I am the greatest advocate of mammograms. I'm a believer in preventative medicine."

Her breast cancer diagnosis was devastating. Annette left the surgeon's office and went to a previously arranged lunch with two girlfriends directly after that appointment.

"I went to lunch, didn't tell those girls, and just shut down for the entire weekend to try and process it. I came home, I live alone, and I shut myself down to try and get my head around it."

Annette had complete faith in her GP and after discussion, she was referred to a surgeon who suggested operating five days later. She had Jersey Boys tickets and asked for an additional week.

"From talking to him, I understood I had no choice. I had less than a week to comprehend it all."

The surgeon recommended a mastectomy and Annette spent 11 days hospital. She recalls her stay as "wonderful", with beautiful floral arrangements arriving daily to the point where the hospital staff were sure they were looking after a superstar celebrity!

Because Annette lived alone, her recovery after discharge was a greater concern. If she and her medical team had known what was to come, they would not have been worried at all. Annette is blessed with the most incredible support network of family and friends who took care of her every step of the way.

"I lived alone, but I was never alone."

Annette's caring friends set up a roster so that someone was always there for her during recovery from surgery, radiation and also throughout her chemotherapy treatment. She had awful side-effects including nausea, vomiting and the loss of hair, finger and toe nails. At some stages, she couldn't eat, but her friends would be there with all types of food and plenty of encouragement. She had friends who would call her every day and others who would just come and sit with her.

In hindsight, Annette feels that she should have let people in a more. Her prior experiences with illness had modelled behaviour of 'soldiering on' during sickness and she fell into the same mindset.

"It's an automatic thing. People ask how you are and you say, 'I'm fine.' You feel like hell, but you aren't going to say that because it makes the other person uncomfortable."

It was a good thing that Annette's friends knew that she would not ask for help and gave it anyway. In fact, she just mentioned that she wanted to install a new kitchen, and without even asking, friends arrived en masse, taking out the old kitchen, prepping it for the installers—she did not need to lift a finger!

Annette discovered the YWCA Encore group through an ad in the paper and she thoroughly enjoyed not only the hydrotherapy and exercise program, but also the new friendships.

It is now four years on and Annette is doing well. She has just finished a year of saying, "Yes!" to every invitation, resulting in an exciting and busy 12 months.

"I might have been independent to the point of stubbornness, but I had good people, good medical care and a lot of time to reflect. I had people around me who supported me whether I wanted them to or not, and they were with me every step of the way."

∾

JENNY

When Jenny was diagnosed with breast cancer, she was a teacher, a divorced mother with two children and an active competitive sportswoman. It was 1990, she was aged just 41, but was no stranger to cancer. Both Jenny's parents had cancer in their fifties and are now in their nineties. When Jenny's mother was diagnosed with breast cancer, she opted for a radical mastectomy and therefore could offer her daughter first-hand advice.

"I couldn't afford to be sick, I didn't want to have chemo or radiation. I just wanted to get this out of my body. I went into surgery on a Wednesday and was back at work the following Monday."

Jenny had a mastectomy and stayed with her mother during recovery. She couldn't pull her hair in a ponytail, do up a button on her skirt or drive, but she managed to teach!

She simply got on with her life and career. Jenny considered reconstruction, but back then the techniques were not as advanced as they are today. She was told that the best option would ruin her back. She thought, "Why would I ruin another part of my body?" and decided against it.

Around nine months later, Jenny was marking some papers when she noticed a lump in her other breast. She saw her oncologist who took a biopsy and sent her for a mammogram which came back as clear. Unfortunately, the biopsy was positive, and the oncologist informed her that it was another primary site in her other breast.

Jenny went in for surgery and had a second mastectomy and they also removed all the lymph nodes. Following surgery, Jenny was prescribed a drug that was originally created to prevent heart attacks in men. Research discovered that the same drug could potentially be helpful in treating women after breast cancer surgery. Jenny was invited to join a trial of Tamoxifen, a drug that is still commonly prescribed, and she continued on that treatment for five years.

"When I stopped taking the Tamoxifen, I felt a bit nervous, thinking this was a crutch. The oncologist said to me after a time, 'You don't need to come back to see me.' But I still felt it would have been good to go for a check-up once a year."

A few years later, Jenny's original oncologist was leaving the hospital and referred her on to the Millennium Institute, Westmead. Her new oncologist referred her to a gynaecological oncologist who was involved in a research project in conjunction with the Familial Cancer Clinic. Jenny contributed blood samples and in 2009, she was contacted by the Clinic regarding findings by a laboratory in Germany that had identified the particular gene responsible for breast cancer from one of her samples. It turned out to be the BRCA1 gene.

When Jenny looked at her family history, it made sense. Her maternal grandmother, four maternal aunts and two paternal great aunts all had some form of gynaecological cancer. With the new information, Jenny chose to have a hysterectomy. Both of Jenny's daughters also tested positive. As a preventative measure, one daughter chose to have a hysterectomy and the other had her ovaries removed.

Other so-called terminal cancers have also existed in Jenny's immediate family and one such relative survived four times longer than expected. He actually kept a diary for his doctors. Another relative is going strong, eleven years after the expected timeframe.

"We are survivors. In my family, if you get cancer, we think of it as an annoyance."

When Jenny joined the YWCA Encore Group, she heard about the breast reconstruction experiences of other women. She was also suffering from considerable neck and shoulder pain due to the weight of her two breast prostheses.

Jenny decided to rethink her previous decision and in 2014, she had a transverse rectus abdominus musculocutaneous flap (TRAM flap) reconstruction of her breasts. Jenny is happy with the result, and also the fact that she has been cancer free since 1991.

"In the 1990s, you had a mastectomy and they sent you home. Nowadays there are such fabulous resources to assist in all aspects of recovery."

❧

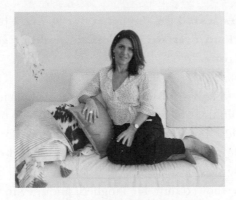

DIANA

With three sons and an accounting business with her husband, Diana's life was incredibly busy. On top of their normal lives, Diana and her husband had also decided to build a new house, and this took several years to complete.

As soon as they moved into their new home, Diana went in for a mammogram. She was 39 at the time and felt guilty that she had not had a mammogram for the past four years. I asked her why she was having screening done at such a young age, and Diana revealed that at age 33, she had two surgeries to remove benign lumps from her breasts. Following these lumpectomies, she was supposed to have annual mammograms. It was a blessing that Diana did resume having mammograms as it was how she discovered her ductal carcinoma breast cancer.

"I knew nothing about breast cancer before this happened to me. I had surgery the following week. I was in shock and had no time to do my own research, so whatever the doctors recommended me to do, I just did it."

Diana had a lumpectomy and in the days after surgery, her medical team arranged a digital tomosynthesis which revealed that her breast had a lot more cancer than originally anticipated. To her horror, she was told that she would need to go back into surgery as soon as possible for a mastectomy.

"The doctors scared the daylights out of me. I just had this big black cloud over my head that wouldn't go away for such a long time."

It took quite a few weeks for Diana to recover. One of the hardest things was explaining it to her youngest son who was only seven at the time. Her two older boys were 18 and 15, so they understood. She tried to keep it simple and told her son that, "The stupid doctor said that Mummy's booby was sick, and he just chopped it off!" He said, "Let me see!" and she showed him. He laughed, and they made it a big joke. Diana felt so much more comfortable after that.

Diana is grateful for the support of her husband and children, and particularly, her Mum who was there throughout her journey.

"My Mum told me, 'Always stay positive, just be positive. You'll be fine.' She constantly drummed it into my head. As annoying as it was at the time, I had to do just that."

The one thing Diana regrets is her decision not to tell anyone what she was going through. It was in part to protect her kids, and also because she was internalising her feelings.

"I kept a lot inside, which really affected me later on. I didn't want to tell people and have to explain myself as it upset me to talk about it. I think it was a very big mistake as I even told my husband, 'Don't tell anybody.' This affected his emotions in a big way. I was upset for a very, very long time and I think that's when the depression and anxiety hit."

Diana did not undergo any further treatment for breast cancer, but this illness was the start of a series of health issues. Six months after surgery, Diana was diagnosed with endometriosis, causing her excruciating pain. This resulted in a hysterectomy and another six-month recovery. The following year, cancer reappeared in the form of melanoma which also required surgery, and then the year after that, Diana had her thyroid removed due to the growth of nodules.

"It has taken many years for me to gain my confidence and love myself again through the aid of my loving husband always telling me, 'You are beautiful no matter what.' Now I am healthy, happy and loving life."

Diana is now 45 and it has been a traumatic six years. She is currently considering breast reconstruction and she feels blessed to have found the group.

"A lovely breast care nurse from the hospital told me about the YWCA Encore Group. It was the best thing she could have ever done for me. We meet up for chats and dinner regularly. I have made new friends for life."

MARIA

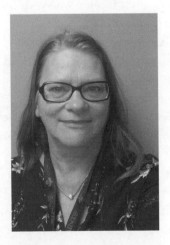

Maria credits a trip to the hardware store for detecting her cancer. She remembers driving into the parking lot of the store and noticing the Breast Screening van. Maria thought to herself, "If that van is still there when I come out, I'm going in there because it's free."

At 46, Maria had no reason to suspect she had breast cancer. It was pure luck that the van was there and that she had time for a screening.

Maria was a laboratory assistant at a local high school, and she took the test just before the Easter school holiday period. When she did not hear from the clinic, she assumed that she was fine and went on a trip. On her return, there was a letter waiting for her assuring her that there was nothing to worry about, but that the clinic wanted her to come in to double check the results.

The day she attended the clinic, Maria found herself with 20 other women who had received the same letter. As each woman went in for her appointment, they would come out smiling saying, "I'm clear! It's all okay." This continued until there were only two ladies left. Maria did a mental calculation of the statistics: one in eight women get breast cancer. She figured that she and the last remaining woman in the waiting room must have a problem.

The first step was a second mammogram with a different machine that focussed in on the suspicious area. For Maria, the position of her cancer was quite high, right at the top of her breast, and it could have easily been missed. The new mammogram magnified the area and Maria noticed that the sonographer was very quiet, asking her to wait to be called for an ultrasound.

By this time, she knew something was up. The ultrasound confirmed that there was an abnormality and Maria was taken to another room for a biopsy.

"The local anaesthetic did not take effect and the biopsy was so painful I had tears running down my face."

The sample was promptly tested and shortly after, a doctor informed her that she needed to have surgery. He proceeded to book her straight into hospital and within two weeks she had a lumpectomy.

Maria is grateful to her friend, a breast care nurse and breast cancer survivor, who gave her some good advice:

"She armed me with a lot of questions. When you see any doctor, there are questions you should ask. Don't be afraid to ask for a second opinion. I was quite open to being guided and the answers made me completely confident in the people looking after me."

During surgery, Maria had a sentinel node removed. It was clear, but as a precaution, she was advised to see both a radiologist and oncologist to discuss her specific case in terms of follow-up treatment.

"The only thing I was worried about, I know it sounds silly because I had a lot of other things to worry about, but my worry was losing my hair. I wasn't worried about being sick, I was worried about losing my hair. I wasn't averse to the chemo, but I was just expressing my concern."

Maria did not need to have chemotherapy because after studying her case, her medical team decided to prescribe radiation therapy and a further surgery to remove her ovaries. Maria's cancer cells had many positive receptors and the doctors thought that her oestrogen production was a trigger, so the removal of her ovaries would solve this problem. Not even six months later, Maria had an oophorectomy and for both operations, she only took two weeks off to recover.

"I think I wanted to be as normal as possible. To make my life stay as normal as it could be with just this one area that was different. I had staples and I was running around a high school! I think, 'Why did I do that?' But anyway, it happened, and it's done."

Maria's breast care nurse suggested she join a support group, but she wasn't ready.

"I didn't want to sit around, talk and feel sorry for myself and indulge in that. That self-pity, I didn't want to go there."

It was only a number of years later, when there were no more medical appointments and she was deemed cancer-free, that the thought of 'flying solo' began to impact her. It was after her final treatment that she started thinking about support.

The friendships in the YWCA Encore Group have helped enormously with this aspect. Maria is so grateful that she happened to see the same newspaper ad as Annette. It was pure chance, a piece of good luck, just like the breast cancer van in the car park.

"Do the best you can, get it over and done with. Just do it."

ZAC

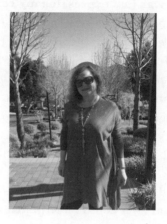

When Zac found a lump near her nipple, she was 29 years old, six months pregnant and running her own optometry business. Zac is a bright and engaging woman whose determination has led to career success and, in terms of her health, was instrumental in obtaining her cancer diagnosis.

Zac went to her obstetrician and her GP who sent her for an ultrasound. The conclusion was that she had a blocked milk gland and that she should massage it. Needless to say, that did not work, as the lump increased in size and was distorting her nipple. She returned to the obstetrician, who said it was nothing and to keep massaging it. Zac felt that it was not right, and she continued to seek answers. She obtained a referral to a surgeon who told her she was overreacting and to go home and have a cup of tea. Zac told him she would feel much better if he took a specimen. She recalls him just "jabbing" her with a needle and sending her away. So, with a surgeon, obstetrician, a gynaecologist and her GP all saying the same thing, Zac put it on the backburner, thinking she was okay.

Eight months later, Zac went back to her home town to visit her mother. By this time her baby girl was five months old. Making a spur of the moment decision, she decided to see her childhood family GP. He examined her and sent her off for an ultrasound and needle biopsy. Two days later, once Zac had returned home (a three-hour drive away), the family GP called asking her to return. She explained that she had only been visiting and asked for the results to be sent to her local GP.

"He said to me, 'I can't believe this is happening. I would have bet my life on it that it was nothing.' And I thought, 'You know what, you bet my life.' He then turned around and said he would send me to a really good surgeon that he would trust with his own health. This is clearly what he should have done to begin with."

It was only Zac's dogged persistence that saved her. She decided to go to a different surgeon who she still sees. He arranged for her to have a bone scan two days later on the Friday, and on Monday she was on the operating table having a lumpectomy.

"I had to stop breastfeeding which was a really difficult thing to do because it was tearing something away."

It is hard enough to deal with breast cancer at any time, but to be diagnosed at one of the few times in a woman's life when your breasts are performing the function of feeding your child, takes the impact to a whole new level. Zac came out of surgery, only to be told that they could not get a clear border and that they could either go back in and cut wider margins or perform a mastectomy. She told them to take the whole breast, and for the second time in seven days, she was back in another surgery.

The operation was successful and Zac, like so many other women, did not have the luxury of taking time to recover. She had a business to run and ended up returning to work as soon as possible. Her chemotherapy began once the incisions were healed and this created new challenges.

> **"When I was having chemo, my brain just wasn't functioning properly. I thought, 'I'm responsible for someone's eye health,' and I just couldn't do it. So, I actually would go in, but I hired a locum to do all the exams for the next five months. It's a real thing, chemo brain."**

Her Mum was "her rock," supporting Zac all the way through her journey. She remembers the oncologist telling her that on her third chemotherapy treatment she would lose her hair and would need to have her wig ready.

> **"After two treatments, my hair was fine. I said to Mum, 'I'm not going to lose my hair, I'll be fine.' And then I had that third treatment and I got up and I couldn't see my pillow for the hair. I decided to take control of it and got my mother and brother to come over and they shaved my hair off. I wasn't going to let it just fall out."**

Zac recovered well and after the recommended six-year clearance period, she had three more babies, all boys. The group is amazed that she breastfed her boys with one breast.

Around 14 years after her lumpectomy, Zac decided she wanted to reclaim her body and investigated reconstruction. Since surgery, she had maintained her routine of an annual mammogram and ultrasound and there were no problems so there would be no obstacles to having her other breast removed prophylactically (preventative procedure) so that she could have a bilateral TRAM Flap reconstruction.

Her surgery went well, and Zac spent 10 days in hospital. On the day she was to be discharged, her surgeon called to inform her that the breast they had prophylactically removed was full of cancer.

> **"It was a completely different type of cancer. The first time it was ductal, and this time it was lobular. I had to go back**

in for surgery and have my lymph glands removed from the right side."

With her lymph glands removed from the left side 14 years ago, Zac now faced having virtually no lymphatic drainage from her arms. When the removed lymph glands were tested, thankfully they were clear. Zac did not need chemotherapy, but her doctor did prescribe radiotherapy, mainly due to the location being close to the chest wall.

Due to her diagnoses, Zac was tested for the BRCA 1 and BRCA 2 genes, but they were not found. However, doctors believe that there is a genetic link to her cancer, one that has yet to be identified. Zac will definitely ensure that her young daughter is tested in her early twenties.

Zac had excellent support from her family and friends. With these people beside her and her positive attitude, Zac was able to handle everything life presented, including the end of her marriage shortly after her second cancer.

Throughout her journey, Zac has adapted to her body changes. In front of her children, she is fine with them seeing and knowing what happened.

"I'm not ashamed of my body, I haven't done anything wrong. I know the people around me love me for who I am, and the state of my breasts does not come into play, it's irrelevant!"

Zac made a full recovery and is cancer-free. She and her children continue to thrive.

"Going back to work quickly kept me occupied. I didn't want to sit at home and be sick. That's just not on. Keeping busy is one of the most important things."

24

MY STORY

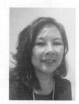

DIAGNOSIS: EXTRA NODAL MARGINAL ZONE LYMPHOMA

For as long as I can remember, I have always felt compelled to find my purpose. My Chinese parents would tell you that my nature is in line with my year of birth—in Chinese astrology, I am a fire horse—independent and always galloping off to discover new horizons.

After moving past childhood fantasies of being a judge or an archaeologist, the one love that persisted was stories. I was a voracious reader and passionate writer of all the characters and adventures conjured up by my overactive imagination.

When choosing my career, I discovered that people would pay me to write! How marvellous! I completed a Bachelor of Arts (Communications) and this became the gateway to an exciting career in marketing, PR, advertising, sales, coaching, and public speaking.

My corporate career transformed into freelance consulting when I decided to have children. My daughter came into the world four weeks early via emergency caesarean. She was black and blue from a 24 labour, hitting her large head against my small hip bones in her attempt to be born.

Perhaps I watched too many romantic comedies, but I had

expected to have that moment when my newborn baby would be placed on my chest, so I could experience the euphoria of instant bonding. The actual moment played out like this: my doctor muttered, "It's a girl," as I watched my baby being whisked away.

I wanted to jump off the operating table and follow her but with a 20 cm (7.9 in) incision in my lower abdomen, I wasn't going anywhere. All I could do was ask questions and the doctors sewing me up were lousy actors. Their reassurances were far from authentic.

My body went into shock and I shook violently and uncontrollably for what seemed like hours. It could have been a reaction to the anaesthetic combined with the panic of not knowing the state of my daughter.

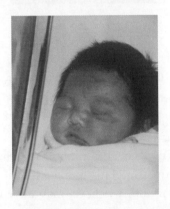

My newborn daughter

Several hours later, I was finally advised that she was badly bruised and suffering extreme jaundice, a condition where there is too much bilirubin. In a premature baby, the immature liver cannot process the bilirubin fast enough and the bruising created an additional load on her tiny body.

The paediatrician told us that if her bilirubin count exceeded 500, my daughter would need a blood exchange transfusion. A good friend went through this exact experience and attributes her constant health battles to this procedure. This knowledge played on my mind and was a future that I did not want for my baby.

There is nothing more frustrating than the feeling of absolute helplessness when the life of a loved one is threatened. Having been both a patient and a parent, for me, being the parent of a sick child was by far the worst. I would have swapped places with my child in a heartbeat.

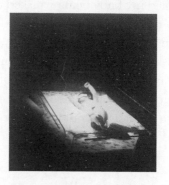

My daughter in phototherapy

For two weeks, I sat by my baby, unable to think straight as I watched her struggle. She was in phototherapy, placed in a shallow box like a plant under growth lights. Her bilirubin count peaked at just under the danger level at 466 and to our relief, day by day, her levels receded to normal.

Five years later, I contracted an innocuous flu virus when I was 14 weeks pregnant with my son. This sparked a series of health issues that wreaked havoc on him and, I believe, may have largely contributed to my cancer diagnosis.

It was one of those viruses that everyone caught. I remember friends and family coughing and sneezing then recovering after around two weeks. When it got to me, unlike everyone else, the virus decided to settle in and a month later I was getting worse instead of better. I lost my voice, and every cough was excruciating painful.

My GP sent me to a respiratory specialist who informed me that my constant coughing had shredded my lungs. My symptoms had caused damage to the tissue in my throat and lungs. Due to my pregnancy, doctors were limited in the types of medication they could prescribe, and I was admitted to hospital for two weeks.

By the time I went home, I had only improved marginally, and I was unwell for my entire pregnancy. I recall taking nine different types of medication. It was a no-win situation—I had to take the medication to get well enough to nourish my growing baby, but what effect was it having on my unborn child?

From the lessons learnt through my daughter's birth, I insisted on having an ultrasound at 35 weeks. It showed that my son's head was already the size of a 42-week old baby and to be honest, I could not wait to get him out!

He was born via planned caesarean four weeks premature, and with the same jaundice as his sister despite avoiding the trauma of labour. We learned later on that the cause was an incompatibility between his mother and father's blood types.

I sat by his humidicrib going through the same helpless emotions for the second time, waiting, watching, wishing there was something I could do but knowing there was not. For those first two weeks in hospital, while every other mother was cuddling their baby, I stared through the plastic humidicrib and could only hold him during breastfeeding.

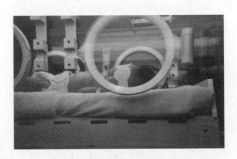

My newborn son in a humidicrib

It was inevitable that there would be consequences for my son, and though he recovered from jaundice, his first six months in the world were very difficult. He was diagnosed with asthma and we spent many sleepless nights listening for any changes to his breathing. I cannot remember how many times we arrived at The Children's Hospital emergency department where they would immediately usher us through and connect him to oxygen and administer Prednisone and Ventolin.

I was grateful that he breast-fed well and resembled a little "Michelin Man," with rolls of fat reminiscent of the Michelin tyre.

company character. During each visit to the hospital, he would lose a kilogram or two and when he came home, his big appetite ensured he gained it back. Getting a blood sample out of those chubby little arms was a huge challenge!

I will never forget one time when we rushed to hospital in the middle of the night as he was struggling to breathe. My son was admitted for a few days as usual, and when I went home to get some clothes, I noticed I had a painful rash developing around my torso. A visit to the GP diagnosed it as shingles. Because it is a derivation of chickenpox, I was not allowed into the children's ward, so his father stayed with him. My daughter had not had chickenpox, so my mother took her away and I was home alone in agony. It was an awful time and the catalyst to take the paediatrician's advice to move to a more temperate climate.

In Sydney, the temperature can be 30°C (86°F) one day, and 19°C (66°F) the next. My son's baby lungs could not cope, and this was a contributing factor to his asthma attacks. We decided to move to the Gold Coast in Queensland, a state that lives up to the marketing slogan "Beautiful one day, perfect the next."

With the change of climate and the addition of chiropractic care and naturopathy, my son's health improved dramatically.

It is difficult to quantify the effect of my prolonged illness and the medication taken during pregnancy, but it would be fair to say that my immune system was severely suppressed as evidenced by the shingles. I was also diagnosed with postpartum thyroiditis and this led to hypothyroidism, a condition I continue to deal with today.

Four years after my son's birth, at age 39, an abnormal pap smear led to a visit to the gynaecologist to explore further. I had a colposcopy. He took a biopsy that was sent away and a few days later I was told that I had CIN3 and at high risk of cervical cancer.

My specialist told me he wanted to perform a Large Loop Excision of the Transformation Zone (LLETZ) to remove all the abnormal tissue. At the time, I felt that he was rushing me into surgery. I really did not want to spend any more time in hospital and asked if I could try some alternative treatments before going down that path. He looked at me with a withering, patronising expression and told me that I would be back because whatever I was going to try would not work.

I left that appointment feeling anxious, wondering if I had made a stupid choice. Research informed me that cervical cancer is a slow growing cancer, however, I was wary because the abnormal cells had developed in the two years since my last pap smear.

Surely anything had to be better than surgery. My naturopath told me of people she had helped in similar situations, so I made the decision to try the alternative path for six months, and if there was no improvement, I would go and have the surgery.

My naturopath put me on a regime of homeopathic tonics and supplements, and though it did not remedy my condition, my overall health undeniably improved. After six months, I decided to go back to be assessed by a different specialist and he recommended that I have the procedure.

I went ahead with the LLETZ and my specialist was happy with the outcome, but my body did not agree. Instead of having my period for a few days a month, I was experiencing the reverse scenario: bleeding all month, with a few days off.

After putting up with it for a few months, I went back to my gynaecologist and he recommended a hysterectomy. He was lovely man with a lilting Irish accent and a dry sense of humour. I remember laughing as he did the math on how a hysterectomy at my age would save me around four years of period bleeding if I added up all the weeks between now and menopause. He then asked me if I had completed my family because if I did not want to have any more children, he may as well take out the "nursery."

I had not planned to have any more children, but the obvious consequence of the procedure meant shutting that door forever.

The doctor's advice was a sensible and logical solution to my health problem, but I remember a moment of hesitation. At the time, I could not articulate why, but looking back, I believe it was the fact that a woman's identity is in part defined by her ability to reproduce and the finality of never being able to do that again was sobering.

I came to terms with what I had to do and booked the procedure. The hysterectomy was problem-free except for my discovery that morphine made me nauseous and violently ill. For the third time, I was opened up through the same scar used for my daughter and son's caesarean births. I sometimes wonder if it would have been more practical to install a zipper down there considering the number of times the same place has been cut open!

Apart from my health issues, this was a very stressful time financially. Due to a desperate need for cash, shortly after my hysterectomy I had to find work and I started consulting to the real estate industry in marketing and sales.

I was supporting the family financially and succeeding at work. My marriage was heading in the opposite direction, and it was during this time that we separated and divorced. Now I was on my own, struggling with debt and paying all the bills on my own. I remember thinking, "What if something happens to me?" My kids would be destitute, and I wasn't going to allow that to happen. The best thing I did was to invest in income protection insurance.

In 2012, I went to the doctor for a regular check-up. She took bloods, examined my breasts and all seemed to be fine. I was 45 and due to my history, she suggested I book in for a mammogram even though the recommended age was 50. I scheduled it for two weeks later and went home.

One week later, I noticed a lump in my breast. It had literally come up out of nowhere and had certainly not been there at my check-up. I returned to the doctor and she was as surprised as I was and arranged an immediate mammogram. There was definitely a problem and I was sent for an ultrasound and fine needle biopsy. The ultrasound was easily done, but the biopsy proved difficult. After five attempts, they gave up. I was referred to a breast surgeon who decided to go in and excise the lump and a lymph node under my left armpit.

Of course, all I could think of was breast cancer. There was so much awareness of breast cancer in the media, and my understanding was that lumps in breasts usually equalled breast cancer. But I consciously tried to avoid the path of worry and fear because I did not yet have a definite diagnosis. Even so, niggling thoughts of losing one breast or both kept popping into my head, but every time it did, I would mentally steer myself in a different direction. Until I knew for sure, I did not want to upset anyone, especially my children who were aged 15 and 10 at the time.

Since the birth of my babies, I attended all of my medical appointments on my own. My family and closest friends lived 1000 km

(620 mi) away, and I did not want to bother anyone else with my problems. It was probably also part of my character makeup that I did not want to ask for help because I thought that I should be strong enough to handle things on my own.

The lumpectomy went well, and I emerged with two new scars. When I returned to the surgeon for the verdict, he asked me if it would be okay if a colleague joined us. My immediate thought was, "this can't be good." He said I was a special case, a rare presentation that he had only seen once in 30 years. I thought, "This is the one time when I do not want to be special." The big reveal was that I definitely had cancer, but not breast cancer, I had lymphoma.

Lymphoma typically presents with swelling in the lymph nodes close to the surface of the body such as the neck, groin or armpits. Because it is a cancer of the lymphatic system, it can also appear in other areas but, as I discovered, it rarely appears in the breast. I asked for the implications, and being a breast surgeon, he said I would have to go and ask a haematologist.

The diagnosis was in some ways a relief. The thought of losing my breasts, was worse than the hysterectomy because as a woman, my breasts formed part of my self-image. Yes, I had cancer, but I was thankful it was not breast cancer.

For various reasons including work and family, I decided to move back to Sydney for treatment. I was lucky to come under the care of Professor Lindeman at the Prince of Wales Hospital.

My PET scan and CT scan confirmed a diagnosis of extra nodal marginal zone lymphoma. I had lumps in my back, my jaw and my hip area. A lump in my back was biopsied and I also had a bone marrow biopsy. If you are wondering what it feels like, imagine being stabbed with a screwdriver so deep it pierces your hip bone. Then it is twisted around to bore out a sample, before being yanked out of your body. Anaesthetic is useless because it cannot numb the bone so out of all the tests I have endured, this one was the worst.

My treatment regime involved chemotherapy, every four weeks for four months and then every three months for two years. The treatment was effective and while I was on it, the lumps did not return.

The main side effects I experienced were extreme fatigue, muscle aches and pains, thinning hair and dry mouth. It did not matter how much water I drank or what I drank, my mouth would always feel dry.

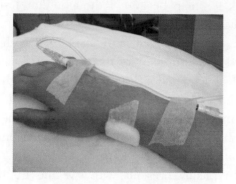

Hooked up for chemotherapy

There were some days I was so devoid of energy that moving off the couch was a big effort. Other days, everything ached. For the first time in my life, I had to respect that my body had limits and when it demanded rest, even my tough mental mindset could not overcome my body's needs.

Another side-effect that I experienced was loss of balance. I had never heard about this and for a long time, I could not work out why I was having problems with one-legged yoga poses and balancing on a bike. Once I did some research, I felt much better knowing that it was a legitimate side-effect and not just me.

"Chemo brain" definitely affected me too. Having a nimble mind is something I value greatly, and I found that chemotherapy made my brain discombobulated. Finding memories was akin to searching for lost items in a thick fog. The mental action of summoning thoughts and words, previously instantaneous, now felt like groping for a light switch in the dark.

This situation was exacerbated by the start of blinding migraines that began in 2013. An MRI showed that my cerebrospinal fluid was thinner than usual and that could perhaps be a contributing factor.

The problem with head issues is the difficulty in diagnosing the cause and treatment. I was referred to a leading neurologist, Dr Granot and he was concerned that I could have lymphoma in the brain. I was sent for a lumbar puncture. This involved lying very still on my stomach while a doctor used a very big needle to draw a sample of fluid from my spine.

I was thrilled to hear that the test came back all clear but unfortunately, the lumbar puncture compounded the problem by causing a post-dural puncture headache (PDPH). This was caused by the leakage of cerebral spinal fluid into the epidural space.

The treatment for this is an Epidural Blood Patch (EDBP). I had to go back for a procedure where they drew blood from my arm, then injected it into the lumbar puncture site in my spine to block the leakage. Unfortunately, the first one did not work, and I had to go back in for a second attempt.

Simultaneous to these treatments, my neurologist began the process of determining which type of medication would help my migraines. I tried around six different medications, but they produced untenable side effects: some made my already foggy brain even worse, some caused dramatic weight gain and did nothing to lessen the pounding in my head.

I was starting to think that I would have to live with this nightmare for the rest of my life without any hope of relief. My neurologist is on the forefront of all new treatments and I was lucky that he was one of the first to use Botox in migraine treatment. The Botox protocol involves 31 injections into the head and neck and it is believed to work by relaxing the muscles that are sensitive to pain.

The treatment did help, and the best part was that it did not create side-effects like those developed by taking medication. I still have this treatment and continue to search for other ways to alleviate the continual pain.

My main concern at my cancer diagnosis was the problem of no income. It took months to negotiate my insurance claim, and during that time I was unable to work, demand letters were arriving too frequently, and my emotional state was hit by the effects of the chemotherapy and the financial crisis. It was my lowest point, drowning in debt, physically weak and emotionally overwrought with no known way out.

I was blessed to have family and friends step up with advice and pathways to resolve a lot of these issues, and eventually pulled myself out of that dark place.

It was a bad year for health issues. I was finding it difficult to walk, experiencing bad pain in my big toes with every step. X-rays showed that the cartilage in my big toes had completely worn away and the pain was being caused by bone rubbing on bone. Why the cartilage in this particular part of my body was affected remains a mystery, but doctors suggested it could have been the chemotherapy, or the autoimmune disease shown in my blood tests as a result of having glandular fever in my twenties. It is impossible to say, but all I can tell you is that the pain was very real.

My GP sent me for cortisone injections which were only mildly effective. She then sent me to an orthopaedic surgeon who looked at my feet and said he could fix it with a bilateral toe fusion. As a shoe lover, I had an enviable collection of spectacular heels. My career had involved many public speaking engagements and I was known for my fabulous shoes. It was part of my identity. The surgery would reduce me to shoes with a 3 cm (1.2 in) heel, ruling out about 80% of my shoe wardrobe—a devastating prospect for any shoe-loving woman.

Surgery became inevitable. I emerged from hospital with 6 cm (2.4 in) wounds and plates with eight screws in each foot.

Until you do not have the use of some part of your body, you do not realise how important mobility is to your daily life. My greatest challenge was taking a shower while keeping both of my bandaged feet dry.

I was able to hobble around but my speed was painstakingly slow. My feet eventually healed, but two years later I broke my right toe and had to have surgery to repair the fracture and the fusion.

And just to keep things interesting, in the middle of all this excitement, I had a terrible pain in my chest and thought I was having a heart attack. An ambulance was called, and the paramedics rushed me to hospital. It turned out to be my gallbladder and within weeks, I lost another vital organ.

During my surgeries and recovery periods, I completed the two-year regime of chemotherapy. In 2015, after six months of remission, my lymphoma returned, and I had to start again with another two years of chemotherapy. I still continue to have my regular checks.

I believe that everything happens for a reason and that my cancer journey has led me back to writing. My past experiences have made me re-evaluate my life and look at what is truly important to me. I now know that my purpose is to make a difference through words.

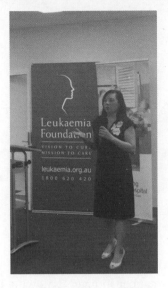

Speaking at a Leukaemia Foundation Function

The greatest lesson I learned through my journey is resilience. Apart from these physical health issues, I have endured financial, relationship and abuse traumas. Just one of these events could have broken me, let alone the cumulative effect of all of them in one lifetime.

Each life challenge builds your resilience for the next bigger challenge. Every time I overcome an emotional or health issue, it makes me stronger. My goal is to learn from the experience and to add the lesson to my repository of knowledge and understanding to help me to become a better me, so that I can fulfil my purpose of positively impacting the world around me.

"Every experience, good and bad, has made me who I am. I've learned that no matter what happens, I can choose how I will respond. I choose to be resilient. I choose to be better, not bitter. I don't ask, 'Why did this happen to me?' I ask, 'What can this help me become?'"

25

FOR THE PATIENT: TACTICS TO SURVIVE AND THRIVE

I HOPE THAT THE STORIES IN THIS BOOK HAVE PROVIDED INSPIRATION and optimism for your cancer journey. Knowing that other people have survived a similar journey to the one you are experiencing can give you the strength, courage and hope to move forward positively.

Inspiration can uplift you immeasurably, but it is the practical knowledge and information that can ease day-to-day challenges that a cancer diagnosis brings.

When I was diagnosed with cancer, I felt like a defective piece of machinery placed on a conveyor belt in a processing plant. I was examined and tested, defective parts were removed, chemicals were added to improve me and at the end they told me I was fixed and to get back to my life.

And if the medical appointments and procedures were not enough to contend with, what about all the other areas of my life?

What was I supposed to do about work? My diary became filled with endless medical appointments instead of work appointments.

How was I going to take care of my children while I was in hospital for surgery? How would my children cope with the knowledge that their mother had cancer? Would they even comprehend what it meant? How did I feel about it? As a single mother, how would I pay the bills if I ended up being unable to work?

What would I tell my family and friends? How would I tell them? What if I died? Would my hair fall out? How sick would I get? Was it curable? Who should I tell?

Did I need a second opinion? I read something about clinics that can miraculously cure cancer. Should I find one of them? Will people be awkward around me and disappear from my life? I have never asked for help. Did I need it and how would I do it without feeling embarrassed or indebted?

These and many more troubling questions raced through my mind in the days after diagnosis. No one amongst my close family and friends had experienced cancer so my knowledge was extremely lacking. I know I am not alone in this respect, despite all the media coverage and fundraising for cancer. This was demonstrated recently when I was at a social function and was asked about the subject of this book.

When I briefly described it, the person enquiring said, "Well you won't find anyone to interview because they are all dead." Yes, this comment was made in the year 2018 by an educated man. My response was, "I have cancer. Am I dead?" It reminded me that despite the growing profile of cancer, many people still associate the big "C" with death.

Looking back, I wish I could have talked to someone or read about someone who had been through a similar experience. I wish I could have learned some real strategies and options available to me that other survivors have used to deal with the impact of cancer in their lives.

From my interviews with all of the people in this book, there are some common themes that have emerged as helpful strategies to minimise the impact of cancer on your life.

1. ASK QUESTIONS

You can ask questions. There is no limit to the number of questions you can ask. There are no stupid questions. No matter how brilliant your surgeon or oncologist, their forte may not be excellent communication. You have them as your specialist because they are extraordinary at their profession, not because they can make small talk or have an incredibly soothing bedside manner. This does not mean that you have to accept every word they say submissively. It is your body that is involved, so you have the right to ask whatever you feel is important.

If you are anything like me, I had no idea what questions to ask. We are lucky to have access to the internet and the ability to research just about any topic on the planet. My suggestion is to feel free to research whatever you want to know, but do not treat that information as gospel. Use Dr Google to learn more about your situation and to help you pose informed questions to your medical team. This way, you will get specific answers to your questions and possible outcomes. A question such as, "What are the known side effects of the drug, Mabthera?" is a much better question than, "What happens when I have chemo?"

2. FIND THE RIGHT MEDICAL FIT

Doctors are human beings. They are highly trained experts, but their advice is based on their personal experience with patients and knowledge gathered from study. It would be ridiculous to think that every doctor knows about every case of your type of cancer that has occurred in the world. Your doctor will give you a best recommendation, but this does not mean that there may not be other opinions to consider. Your first recommendation may well be the best option and you may choose to take it, but if something does not sit well with you, you have every right to seek another opinion.

With other professions, we think nothing of getting a few quotes before choosing which provider will get the job. If your car needs a tune-up or a specific service, it is considered due diligence to get at least three quotes before determining which you will use. Why then, do we treat doctors' recommendations as indisputable fact?

Doctors are not omnipotent, they are highly educated and skilled human beings. Humans are not infallible and no two are alike. Two doctors may have the same specialist title but their opinion and recommended treatment plan for a patient may not be the same. One doctor may have experienced positive outcomes with a particular treatment, while the other may have undertaken research in a particular field and may recommend a different treatment. Any number of variables in skill, education, experience and knowledge can exist between professionals with the same accreditation.

Many of the stories in this book testify to the fact that it is imperative that you trust your instincts when proceeding with treatment. You will remember reading about Ken, diagnosed with Non-Hodgkin's Lymphoma who was booked in for surgery but cancelled because he felt uneasy. Further investigations with a different doctor supported his decision. Surgery was avoided, and chemotherapy treatment was prescribed instead.

Another story that comes to mind is Zac who, without seeking the advice of several specialists, would not have discovered her diagnosis of breast cancer. Who knows what would have happened if she had believed the first doctor she saw, who told her there was nothing to worry about? Her breast cancer would have continued to spread, and Zac's positive outcome could have ended up very differently had her cancer had not been detected as early.

You have the right to choose. If you are satisfied with your medical team, believe in them and follow their advice. If you are concerned, discuss your thoughts with trusted family or friends and seek out opinions from other professionals until you have complete confidence in your team and feel 100% satisfied with your treatment plan.

3. DEALING WITH EMOTIONAL TURMOIL

From the moment of diagnosis, it is completely normal to feel that your world has been turned upside down. Everything you thought about your life: plans for the future, your job promotion, the dream trip you booked, the new house you have just purchased, the private school that your child has been accepted into, the wedding you have arranged…all of it is threatened in an instant.

Not only do you suddenly need to become a cancer expert and decide on treatment that will affect the rest of your life, you also have to work out how it will affect every other area of your life. You may feel overwhelmed, your carefully laid plans now collapsing all around you. What can you do to avoid falling into a bottomless pit of despair? The stories you have read show you the different ways people coped with the emotional impact of their diagnosis.

i. Feel Your Emotions

Your emotions and feelings are valid. You might feel anger at how unfair it is that you have cancer. Your initial shock and numbness may give way to hopelessness and depression. You may be scared or anxious. You may feel worry for the future of your family. Whatever you feel, acknowledge your emotions as real. Resist the urge to push them inside while putting on a brave face. This was something that was very hard for me to do as I had spent a lifetime perfecting this method of dealing with problems. You may be the same, always looking happy and together on the outside, but actually hiding your true emotions in a locked box on the inside.

Unfortunately, this is a flawed strategy. Cancer is a journey and your emotions will rise and fall along the way. Many interviewees said that they regretted not speaking out truthfully during their cancer journey, thinking that they were being stalwart, or protecting their family from their pain and fear, when it often had the opposite effect of causing more angst and worry.

Help yourself and your loved ones by communicating your true feelings. Verbalising your emotions is a way for you to process your emotions and the simple act of sharing your burden will help lighten your load and provide another perspective on your circumstances.

Dealing with emotions throughout your journey will keep you in a healthier mental state. Being honest with your support team helps them to provide what you truly need rather than what they think you need.

ii. Find a Guide

Your cancer journey will take you through some rough emotional terrain. You may go through some dark forests and feel that you cannot even see past the tree in front of you. You may sink into a deep valley of despair. A positive result from a test may have you shouting from the highest mountain. Complications or a new diagnosis may leave you numb, in shock, unaware of anything around you.

I've met many cancer survivors who found someone amongst their friends and family who they could unreservedly open up to in order to deal with their emotions.

Perhaps it is someone who loves you unconditionally and can hear you and provide sage advice and guidance. If you have that person to lean on, keep them close beside you on your journey.

You might connect better with someone who has been through their own cancer journey. Remember the story of Rex whose brother-in-law had survived the same prostate cancer diagnosis some years before? Being able to discuss the emotional impact with someone who understood completely what it felt like to deal with the effects of this disease made a big difference to him psychologically and emotionally.

iii. Get a Counsellor

For me, the best thing I did was to find a psychologist, someone who I could speak to without fear of consequences. Her only objective was to help me to heal and to deal with the chaos that had swallowed up my life.

If you are not sure who you can speak to, seek out the many organisations and institutions who provide counselling services for cancer patients and their families. The Cancer Council and Leukaemia Foundation have wonderful support staff and counselling services available. There are also organisations such as CanTeen for teenagers and their families dealing with cancer, and Camp Quality for children with cancer and their families. Many church and religious groups also provide counselling services.

iv. Seek Support Groups

For some, becoming part of a support group is a wonderful way to connect with other people who have been through similar experiences. Search the internet for local groups in your area. Use social media and in particular, Facebook to identify groups you can join and people you can connect with. No matter how much your family and friends love you, it can make all the difference to share your feelings, specific issues and questions with someone who has personally walked the same path.

Reading stories is another great way to find out how other people have handled their cancer diagnosis and treatment. Two stories that illustrate how beneficial support groups can be are the ones in this book about Adam and also the Encore Group.

For Adam, finding the Head and Neck Cancer Survivors group helped him to connect with other people who had suffered similar cancer diagnoses and treatment. He contributed to growing the group to reach and support many others.

The Encore Group women similarly expressed the camaraderie that exists between them due to the shared experience of breast cancer. Even though they have completed the program that brought them together, they still keep in touch and meet up regularly.

Only you can decide what type of emotional support you need for your journey. One way is not better than another, the best choice is the one that works for you.

4. CHOOSE A PRIMARY SUPPORT PERSON

Throughout your cancer journey, you may wish to nominate one person, perhaps a partner, parent, sibling or good friend who is fully informed of your medical history and current status and treatment. It is a great idea to have this person attend medical appointments with you, not only for the emotional support, but also for practical organisational assistance. This primary caregiver can help you with the following important tasks:

i. Lending You Brain Power

With your brain flooded with who knows how many emotions, and your body likely to be recovering from surgery or your latest round of chemotherapy, your ability to think clearly is likely to be sub-par. When you are sitting in your specialist's rooms and he tells you he needs to go back in and remove more tissue to get wider margins, it really helps to have someone there asking questions on your behalf, because you have likely gone into disbelief at having to go through that all over again.

Many people interviewed said that having someone with them was invaluable. The shock of the news overloaded their brains and they reported being ever so grateful that someone was there to ask the pertinent questions.

ii. Helping to Keep Your Treatment On Track

Depending on the effects of your cancer and treatment, you may or may not be feeling well enough to schedule all your appointments or to get yourself to those appointments. Your support person can ensure you do not have to worry about the details, so you can focus on things that will help the healing process.

The other thing they can help you do is to keep a record of test results, appointment outcomes, important information provided by your medical team, medication schedules and recovery instructions. You or your support person can keep a file that can be easily referenced. This is particularly useful if you are referred to a new specialist and it is a quick and easy way to brief them on your medical history.

One of the best records I have seen was kept by Bob and Helen. When I interviewed Bob, it was easy to remember what happened as they had recorded every appointment, medication and outcome over the course of Bob's journey.

iii. Assisting You During Recovery

At some stage during your cancer treatment, there will be a recovery period from surgery or treatment. This will be different for every person, depending on the type of cancer and the effects of your treatment. You may be one of those people who breezes through this part with little need for assistance, or you may find yourself discharged from hospital, unable to bathe yourself. Whatever your circumstances, accept the support you need to get on the road to recovery. Whether it is family or friends taking turns to help you, or a nurse who visits regularly, do not be too proud or embarrassed to accept their kindness.

5. GATHER YOUR TRIBE

When your friends and family find out you have cancer (the grapevine is still an incredibly fast way for news to travel!), people will react in different ways. As you will have discovered through reading the previous chapters, some people will be positive, supportive and offer tangible assistance. Others will feel awkward, say a few platitudes, and may even disappear from your life. It is not always because they do not care. It may be that they do not know how they can help you or what they should do.

There will be other well-meaning people who will ask you if you have tried any number of miracle cancer cures. I still have people who tell me that they saw a new amazing drug on the TV last night and I should check it out. I generally just nod and say thank you as I understand that it is said out of love, but in reality, I'm thinking, "My specialist is on the cutting edge and if there was another drug with greater efficacy, he would prescribe it."

Everyone reacts according to their own bank of knowledge created from their own past experiences with cancer. The important thing here is not to worry about those who are not positive and supportive. Let them go. Gather the ones who will be there for you, who bring positivity and hope to your life, who do not expect any payback but give from their heart. Find the people who are uplifting, who make you laugh and feel light, focussing on you as a person, and not the cancer.

Remember the story of Annette, the woman who lived alone but was never alone. She had a wonderful tribe who surrounded her with practical and emotional support throughout her breast cancer journey.

You do not need any negativity or bad attitudes around you. Your body is already in a battle for health and it needs every weapon in the armoury to win. Find a tribe of like-minded people to buoy you up.

6. PRACTICAL PLANNING

Much of the emotional trauma caused by a cancer diagnosis is related to the practicalities of how to maintain the commitments of normal life while dealing with cancer treatment. Depending on your regime, you many need extended time off work, children that need to be cared for, arrangements that need to be altered. Plans need to be made and put into place to ensure things are taken care of when you are in surgery, treatment and recovery. Here are some important things to think about:

i. Get Informed

Planning requires information. Once your regime is set, ask your medical team the questions that will allow you to understand what is involved in your treatment. Obviously, there may be issues that will cause changes, but they can tell you the usual outcomes if all goes as expected. If you are having surgery, ask how long you are likely to be in hospital. Ask about recovery periods and whether there will be restrictions of movement or certain physical tasks. Check on the side-effects of your medication. If you are having chemotherapy, ask what the usual side-effects and recovery periods tend to be with most patients. Ask for the expected duration of your treatment. By finding out exactly what is involved, you will be able to make arrangements with your work colleagues, alter plans for the period of your recovery and if necessary, arrange care for your children.

ii. Accept Assistance

Don't do what I did. When anyone asked me how I felt, I would say I was fine. I was that person who other people asked for help. I prided myself on being mentally tough and resilient and thought that asking for help made me seem weak.

I also did not want to bother friends and family—I did not want their pity or sympathy, nor did I want to feel their well-meaning judgement. Most importantly, I did not want to worry or burden them with what I saw as my problem. This was ridiculously stupid of me and I wish I had accepted the generous offers I received.

Sometimes, helping you through this period is the best way that people can show their love and care. Allow them to assist you, do not let your self-image, or "what people think" hinder your recovery.

What I and the people in this book have discovered is that people want to help. There is a joy in giving that is more satisfying and fulfilling than receiving. By not accepting their kind offers, I was denying people the opportunity to process their emotions about what was happening and also to feel the satisfaction of doing something good.

The greatest gift can be a friend who offers to bring your wife to hospital because she does not drive, as in the case of John and Margaret. It can be offering to pick up your children from school and taking care of them when you are too sick to get out of bed as Nina's parents did. Not having to worry about the small but important stuff will give you peace of mind and the strength to focus on recovery. It also gives your friends and family a tangible way to help you.

iii. Be Prepared

Nobody owns tomorrow. Being positive and expecting the best possible outcome is key to survival but as we all know, the unexpected can happen. One of the things I heard the most from all of the people that I interviewed was that they were worried about what would happen to their children and family if the worst should happen.

It is impossible to be emotionally prepared for the death of a loved one, but it is possible to alleviate their pain by having all of the legal documentation in place just in case. Ensure that you have the following documents drawn up or updated to reflect your current circumstances and wishes. These may vary according to where you live, and you will need to check the specific requirements in your location. In Australia, the documents that you need to have in place are:

Last Will and Testament
This is a legal document recording who you would like to receive your assets after you die. It can also record your wishes regarding guardianship of your children.

Power of Attorney / Enduring Power of Guardianship
This document appoints your nominated person to make decisions on your behalf if you are no longer able to make them for yourself.

Advanced Care Directive / Living Will
This document records your wishes for your future medical care.

Gather your important documents such as your birth, marriage, divorce and citizenship certificate, bank account information, investment portfolio, government institution details, loan information, passport, will and social media account details. Keep them in a safe place and inform your trusted person of the location.

With this practical and important planning in place, you can have peace of mind, knowing that if things go wrong, all of your affairs are in order and your wishes will be carried out. This can alleviate your anxiety and allow you to focus on the important job of healing.

7. TREATMENT TRAUMA

Depending on your current state of health and your treatment plan, you may or may not be affected by side-effects. For some, side-effects are a non-issue. For others, the side-effects are worse than the actual disease. Ask your medical team for the most common side-effects of the treatment you are undergoing to get some idea of what you might experience.

The National Cancer Institute website provides a comprehensive list of cancer treatment side effects:

- Anaemia
- Appetite Loss
- Bleeding and Bruising (Thrombocytopenia)
- Constipation
- Delirium
- Diarrhea
- Swelling (Oedema)
- Fatigue
- Fertility Issues in Boys and Men
- Fertility Issues in Girls and Women
- Hair Loss (Alopecia)
- Infection and Neutropenia
- Lymphedema
- Memory or Concentration Problems
- Mouth and Throat Problems
- Nausea and Vomiting
- Nerve Problems (Peripheral Neuropathy)
- Pain
- Sexual Health Issues in Men

- Sexual Health Issues in Women
- Skin and Nail Changes
- Sleep Problems
- Urinary and Bladder Problems

It is important to note that side-effects can vary from person to person, even when having the same treatment. You may not experience any of these symptoms, but I believe it is important to be aware of what may happen. When I began my treatment regime, I wondered why I kept bumping into things and bruising badly. It was a long way down the track of my cancer journey before I was informed that these were side-effects of the treatment.

If you are already on your cancer journey and you are experiencing some of these side-effects, go ahead and find out if it is a common result of the drugs you are taking, and research the best ways to alleviate these symptoms.

If you have just been diagnosed, it is good to be generally aware, but there is no need to panic that you will be struck down with all of these side-effects. As you will have read, some of the people in this book, such as Lou, experienced minimal side-effects whereas other people, such as Annie, battled through multiple health issues as a result of her treatment.

Just remember that you are unique, and that no one can definitively predict how treatment will affect you. The important thing is to understand your treatment and if you do suffer from side-effects, then immediately talk to your medical team and work on a solution to the problem.

Thit's story is one where her chemotherapy treatment was so potent that it knocked out her entire immune system and white cell count. Through consultation with her oncologist, they were able to change her treatment protocol so that she could continue.

Do not put up with pain or side-effects with the attitude that it is just part of the process. Speak up and ask for solutions, as Thit did. Doctors do not have telepathy. You need to tell them what is happening and ask for help. Sometimes there may not be a way they can lessen the side-effects and you may need to consider other options. I urge you to seek solutions. If you do not feel well enough, ask your tribe or support team to assist with research. Find out what other people have done to cope with the side-effects and put their knowledge to use.

8. MIND MATTERS

Doctors are trained to look at problems with our physical body and to fix them. Specialists are experts in specific parts of the body. The human body is an incredibly complex system controlled by the brain, which is often considered as separate to the body.

Do the thoughts in our brain affect our physical body? Does it make a difference to the health of our body if our mental attitude is positive or negative, or if our emotions are happy or sad?

It only takes an internet search to pull up multiple research findings from institutions as well-respected as the Mayo Clinic and Harvard University to prove the difference that a positive attitude can make. The placebo effect is the simplest proof that belief can create positive change.

In *The Healing Self*, a book by Dr Deepak Chopra and Dr Rudolph E. Tanzi, both pioneers in their respective fields of integrative medicine and genetic neurological disease, these two major influencers discuss the whole system approach.

According to Chopra and Tanzi (2018), "Nature doesn't recognise human-made categories. Body and mind are one domain, every organ, tissue, and cell works toward the same goal: sustaining life."

The mind is an integrated part of the body and automatically controls all our vital functions. Does it not follow that anxiety and stress in the mind would affect the body?

Chopra and Tanzi note that the body is actually under dual control. We can intervene and disrupt the automatic system by consciously making choices that can either benefit or hinder our well-being. We only need to look around at major societal issues such as obesity or addictions to know that we can easily interfere with optimal health choices through poor eating choices or substance addictions.

They also pose that emotions such as hopelessness, worry, low self-esteem, loneliness, bad relationships and lack of purpose are, by virtue of the body mind connection, affecting our bodies and disrupting our whole-system goal of sustaining life.

In the same way as our negative thoughts can impact our body and mind adversely, so can our positive thinking and good choices assist in improving our health. Every person in this book has embraced a positive mindset and it appears that has played a key role in their ability to survive and to thrive.

There are a number of ways you can help yourself to positively intervene and help your whole system to heal. Here are some methods that have helped others to survive their cancer journey:

i. Meditation

A study by Barbara L. Fredrickson, a psychology researcher at the University of North Carolina, revealed that people who meditate daily display more positive emotions that those who do not. Three months after the experiment was over, the people who continued to meditate displayed increased mindfulness, purpose and decreased symptoms of illness.

I have personally practiced daily meditation for a few years now and can testify to improvement in all of those areas. There are many different types of meditation methods available and you may want to explore the various options to find the one that you feel is the most beneficial. I have found the collaboration between Oprah and Deepak Chopra at Chopra Center Meditation to be a great fit for me.

Search online to discover guided meditations, music meditations and many apps for your phone that make different styles and lengths of meditation easy to access anytime.

ii. Journal or Blog

There is something both therapeutic and tangible about writing things down. A personal journal can be a private place to write down whatever you experience and feel without fear or filter. Let your thoughts flow freely onto the page. I can type much faster than I can write, particularly if it needs to be legible, but I still put pen to paper for my journal. There is something visceral about the process and I imagine the act of handwriting as unburdening my mind and allowing the tangle of thoughts in my mind to move through my hand and onto the paper in any order.

When your worries and feelings are on paper, it moves them to a more objective place where you can see them rather than them being hidden away and roaming wherever they choose in your mind.

Think about opening the refrigerator and realising that you have run out of milk. You are not going shopping until tomorrow, but you need to remember to buy milk. As you go through your day, milk pops into your head and you re-remind yourself that you need to buy milk. You finally get to the store the next day, fill your basket with all sorts of necessary items and impulse purchases, arrive home and realise that you forgot the milk.

Let's change the scenario and imagine that the first time you realised you needed to buy milk, you wrote it down on a shopping list. From that moment on, you did not have to think about it again until you were standing in the store and looking at the list. You had transferred it to another place and freed up your mind to get on with other tasks.

It is a simple analogy, but I believe a similar process occurs when you journal. It relieves your mind from the effort of dealing with worries and thoughts bouncing around your mind randomly. During treatment, eliminating as many unnecessary worries and negative thought patterns as possible leaves room for the positive and healing thoughts that will help your cancer journey.

Writing down positive results and uplifting connections and experiences will also help to reinforce the good that is coming into your life. You might have heard about the benefits of keeping a gratitude journal, writing down something you are grateful for each day. Take the examples of Rex who, on a daily basis asks, "What is the best thing that happened to you today?" and Thit, who kept a journal throughout her cancer journey and wrote down the answer to the question, "What is the blessing that I have today?"

The other positive benefit in writing down your thoughts is that it activates another part of your brain. There have been many studies done on memory and comprehension and educators believe that hearing and reading information brings knowledge into our minds to process. We think about these new ideas and can formulate our views.

But it is only when we verbalise or write these thoughts down in our own words, that the magic happens. We activate different parts of the brain that cause us to evaluate those thoughts and process them before we write them down. In this way, journaling can help you to process the overwhelm of thoughts, worries and emotions that can swamp you throughout your cancer journey.

Blogs are a public way to share your journey. You may or may not feel comfortable with sharing your raw emotions and details in a public forum, but it can be a great way to keep your friends and family aware of what is happening so that you do not have respond to many phone calls and messages explaining the status of your progress again and again. Choose carefully what you wish to share and what you want to keep private. Once something is posted online, it tends to stay in cyberspace forever so keep this in mind.

You could start up a blog page, or you may choose to use social media to post updates. Sarah created a wonderful blog to keep their wide circle of international friends and family aware of their bus adventures and Catur's progress. Before the days of social media, Aaron found it very therapeutic to write a regular email update on Ben and Ella. His email list grew to over 60 people as friends and families appreciated the opportunity to keep informed.

iii. Laugh

Laughter is the best medicine. The truth of this well-known saying is supported by a plethora of medical studies. Many credit Norman Cousins, global peacemaker, recipient of a UN peace medal, hundreds of awards and nearly 50 honorary doctorate degrees, for being instrumental in spreading the knowledge about laughter's positive impact on health. Diagnosed with an incurable disease and only months to live, he embarked upon a regime of Vitamin C injections and laughter. In his book "Anatomy of an Illness," Cousins documents how over the course of two years, he was completely cured.

Laugh with friends, watch funny movies, read books and jokes that make you belly laugh. When we laugh, the entire brain is activated, and feel-good endorphins are secreted. These beta-endorphins can release pain.

A study by Dr William B Stean, medical doctor and professor at University of Atlanta, showed that laughter increases the levels of interferon gamma (IFN) in the body that stimulates immunoglobulin, B-cells, T-cells and NK cells. These are part of the immune system and the first lines of defence against cancer and tumour growth (2009).

Consciously bring laughter into your daily routine to improve every area of your life. Sharing laughter is beneficial emotionally, physically and mentally and builds stronger relationship bonds.

iv. Be Positive

There can be no doubt that a positive attitude plays a vital role in cancer survival. Every story in this book tells of the importance of being positive about recovery and surrounding yourself with encouraging and supportive people. It is a normal human reaction to experience shock, numbness, sadness and even grieving over the loss of function or attributes that we previously took for granted.

Use meditation to calm your mind, journal to help process your feelings and find a way to make play and laughter a regular part of your life. These things can help to lift you out of dark places, but the key is to create a positive mindset about the successful outcome of your treatment.

You can decide how you want to view your cancer diagnosis. You could see it as a tragedy or an unfair curse that has come into your life. If you live in that space and choose it to form your attitude, then it probably will be. As we have established, your mind controls your body's whole system, so your negative thoughts must have an effect on your body.

A great example of choosing a positive rather than a negative outlook is Vi. Only ten days from death, she made the decision to be positive and to surround herself with uplifting people. She was so determined that this was required for her recovery that she was willing to forgo visitation by close friends and family if they could not adopt this mindset. She not only recovered but is now thriving and doing amazing things for the cancer community.

Summon your willpower and resilience to build your positive

mindset because it will be your shield to get you through the ups and downs of your cancer journey.

v. Become Resilient

Depending on your previous life experience, resilience might be a new trait you are learning to develop. For others, it is like an old friend that has kept you moving forward.

Resilience is that ability to recover from trauma, adapt to change and to persist in the face of adversity. Developing it is just like building muscle tone. The first time you lift those weights, you feel like you will never be able to do more than one set of repetitions. If you continue training, soon you can do two sets, then three. If you keep it up, your muscle tone will strengthen and grow. You will be able to do more repetitions and lift heavier weights.

Resilience can be built in a similar way. Everyone faces problems and difficulties throughout their lives. The key is to learn from every experience so that you are better equipped to handle future challenges. By developing and growing in knowledge and wisdom, you will build a greater resilience when traumas enter your life.

Carl's story is an excellent example of using the resilience he learned as an elite athlete to power him through his incredibly difficult cancer journey.

Renae credits the resilience she developed through her cancer journey to helping her and her husband Rick to cope with their son Leo's open-heart surgery just days after his birth.

If you have faced previous life challenges and have become resilient, then you know that cancer is another experience you can get through. This experience will continue to develop a greater level of resilience that will serve you well moving forward.

9. EXTRAS

As you have read in previous chapters, you do have choices about the actions you will take to support your cancer journey. Your medical team is there to destroy the cancer that is inside your body. Beyond that, it is up to you to decide what else you will do to give yourself the best possible outcome. Here is a summary of some of the things that the wonderful people in this book have used to help them to survive and thrive.

i. Get Outside

So much of our cancer journey is spent in hospitals, doctors' rooms, oncology wards, intensive care wards, pathology centres and radiology clinics under artificial fluorescent lighting and in closed air-conditioned rooms.

When you feel well enough, get out into nature. Feast your eyes on a beautiful mountain or ocean vista, breathe fresh pure air, bathe in sunlight and absorb Vitamin D. Connect to the earth's energy by grounding yourself. Take your shoes off and be barefoot, drawing in the earth's electrical charges. It can improve sleep and reduce inflammation. Being outdoors can boost your creativity and memory, ease stress and anxiety.

ii. Eat Wisely

Even though you may feel out of control, the one thing you can still make decisions about is the food that you eat. As the saying goes, you are what you eat. When you have cancer, it becomes more important than ever to give your body the optimal opportunity to heal and that means making good choices about the food you consume.

It is a scientifically proven fact that too much sugar is bad for anyone, and there is evidence, as discovered in a study by Dr Lorenzo Cohen of the University of Texas Anderson Cancer Centre, that some cancers are fuelled by sugar (2016). You have likely heard that many of our fruits and vegetables contain pesticides and chemicals and that packaged foods contain additives and preservatives.

Many people in this book have made the decision to eliminate sugars, chemicals and processed food in their quest for the best possible outcome. They have made choices to eat fresh, organic wholefoods. A great way to access this type of produce is at farmers' markets, where you can purchase produce directly from the farmer, knowing it is freshly harvested.

If this is not possible, look for fruit and vegetables that are certified organic. There are a growing number of health food stores sprouting up around the world as we gain a greater awareness about the benefits of good food choices.

This will ensure that you are not ingesting any harmful chemicals that will only add to the load of toxins that your body has to eliminate.

iii. Supplement

Some people I interviewed swear by the difference that supplementation has made to their cancer recovery. Helen, who is a remarkably fit and healthy 74-year-old, has been cancer free for 26 years and attributes her wellness, in part, to the supplement regime recommended by her naturopath.

Linda found essential oils and in particular, frankincense, to be a wonderful aid to recovery. It has been used for thousands of years as a disease fighting anti-inflammatory oil. Catur has found cannabis oil to be his most effective treatment, while Graham uses many different supplements including high doses of Vitamin C infusions, Vitamin B12, probiotics and enzymes.

Some members of the medical fraternity say that there is no scientific evidence for the efficacy of supplements, but if you are compromised with cancer, then it is certainly worth investigating supplementation and deciding for yourself whether it is an option for you.

iv. Exercise

Exercise is definitely a key factor in the recovery of many of the people in this book. Sharon, a woman who has been through numerous health issues, is a firm believer that exercise helped her to recover following her rare cervical cancer. Mark is also a strong advocate for the benefits of exercise and fitness.

Depending on the effect of your treatment, exercise may be difficult, but try to move your body—even a slow walk is beneficial. According to the Cancer Council, exercise during treatment can help to manage side-effects, speed up your return to normal activities and improve your overall quality of life. Have a look at their website for videos and information on recommended exercise during and after your treatment. You can also talk to your medical team and they may refer you to a physiotherapist to assist you.

v. Therapies

There are numerous other therapies that cancer survivors have used on their cancer journeys. The creation of the Chris O'Brien Lifehouse, alongside the Royal Prince Alfred Hospital in Sydney, demonstrates the growing medical support for the place of natural therapies in the healing of cancer patients. Art therapy, counselling, reflexology, chiropractic, physiotherapy, yoga, qi gong, oncology massage and acupuncture are all regarded as therapies helpful in aiding recovery, and ongoing in maintaining a balanced and healthy mind and body.

I encourage you to explore these and other therapies to find the ones that work to help you to survive and thrive.

From the stories in this book, you will have discovered that there is no single way to handle a cancer journey. If there is just one thing that you take from this book, I hope it is the confidence to trust your instincts. Learn from what others have done and find the options that work for you.

26

FOR FRIENDS AND FAMILY: HOW TO PROVIDE MEANINGFUL SUPPORT

WHAT DO YOU DO WHEN YOU FIND OUT THAT SOMEONE YOU KNOW HAS cancer? Does it make you worried about what to say to them? Do you avoid seeing them because you do not want to be in an awkward conversation? Do you want to offer your sincere concern without sounding trite? What is the best way to help without intruding? How do you offer meaningful support that can genuinely make a difference?

These are the questions that many people ask when they hear about a cancer diagnosis. From discussing the subject of support with all the people in this book, I felt that it was important to include a guide to the 'Do's and Don'ts' when you want to give meaningful support.

1. WHAT CAN YOU DO?

Yes, I have cancer. No, I have not been taken over by aliens and become a cancer being. I am the exact same human being that you have always known. It just happens that I have cancer and I am fighting it with everything I can.

There is no need to treat me differently. I still laugh at the same things and enjoy doing the same things we have always done together, even though some of them may be a bit difficult to do for a while. I understand that you may feel awkward talking about your next hiking trip knowing that I cannot go with you, but please go ahead and chat. You do not need to tiptoe around me. Just be your normal self. I want as much 'normal' as I can have around me. Include me in group chats on social media. It makes me feel human and part of the world when my reality is tubes coming out of my body and drugs going in.

2. WHAT CAN YOU SAY?

I know you love me, that you care and are truly concerned about my prognosis. Please do not ruin it with hollow platitudes. When I am waiting on the results of my PET scan, I do not need to hear, "Oh, you'll be fine." When I am bald and wearing a headscarf, my eyes sunken and my skin grey, I really do not need you to say, "You look great!" I have mirrors and eyes.

If you hear about a new cancer breakthrough on the news, you do not need to phone me immediately to insist that I fly to another continent to apply for a new trial program. I might be getting my first decent night's sleep for several weeks or coping with some nasty chemo side-effects.

I have sought out the best specialists in the particular type of cancer I have and if a medical breakthrough is available to me, I trust my medical team to be onto it. I do, however, appreciate the sentiment and if you have something exciting to share, please tell me or my support people or send me an email so I can investigate.

I know you might feel awkward about having a conversation with me, avoiding the obvious like an elephant in the room. Please just relax and let the conversation flow as it normally would. There is no reason not to talk about cancer in honest and real terms. Rather than worrying about what to say, think more about being a supportive friend or family member who is there to listen. Instead of feeling the need to say something and have it come out of your mouth sounding like a cliché, ask sincere questions such as, "How is your current treatment going?" and, "Is there any task or errand I can help you with?" Offer to be a sounding board or shoulder to lean on and to listen without judgement or advice. Sometimes we just need to be heard. Give me a hug. Research shows that a proper deep hug is nurturing and a powerful way of healing.

3. HOW CAN YOU SHOW YOUR SUPPORT?

There are so many ways to show your support. From the stories in this book, you will have read the many ways that support has been graciously given and received. By far the most universally appreciated assistance was when the tasks of daily living were taken care of by friends and family.

Here is a summary of helpful things you can do. Co-ordinate appropriate times and specifics with me or my support person.

i. Child Care

Help me with picking up my children, taking them to school and to extra-curricular activities. Babysit when both parents need to be at medical appointments or at the hospital.

ii. Meals

Healthy, home-cooked meals are really appreciated. After a long day at work, then a hospital visit, it is a relief to come home and eat a wholesome meal, not having to worry about cooking or the awful prospect of eating more fast food.

iii. Household

Simple chores such as cleaning and gardening make a real difference. A messy home and garden beds full of weeds just add to our burden so taking care of these tasks is enormously valued.

iv. Transport

During treatment, it is not always possible to drive. You can offer to drive me to medical appointments and treatments. I will enjoy your company and be thankful for your support.

v. Time

Offer to spend time with me. I will tell you if I am not up to it, but when I am, it is wonderful to have your company to watch a silly movie with me when I am stuck on the couch. Maybe we could go outdoors and breathe the fresh air.

vi. Love and friendship

Knowing you truly care means a lot to me. I appreciate when you listen to me without judgement when I need to work through my feelings and words tumble out of my mouth. Hug me deeply as it restores my mind and body.

Please do not disappear when my treatment is finished. I might find it difficult to adjust to life. This can be a hard part of my cancer journey. I have been taken off the merry-go-round of medical appointments and am now standing still, working out how to move forward. I still need to know that you care and that you are there for me.

vii. Donate

If cancer has caused me financial difficulties, you can donate supplies or money to help ease my distress.

viii. Fundraise

If cancer has affected my family's ability to earn an income, I may be in extreme difficulty. Fundraising can help to take the financial stress out of an already devastating situation.

Meaningful support is different for every person. If you truly want to support me. Communicate honestly and willingly with me. Take the time and effort to discover how I am really feeling and be genuine in your offer of assistance. This will allow me to open up and tell you what I would appreciate the most.

27

FOR THE PRIMARY SUPPORT PERSON:
HOW TO COPE AS A CAREGIVER

ONE OF THE MOST COMMON AREAS OF DISCUSSION AMONGST ALL THE people in this book was their concern for the impact that their cancer diagnosis had on their spouse, partner, parents and children. Many interviewees talked about how they were more worried and concerned for their loved ones than they were for themselves.

This chapter aims to provide appreciation for the support person of the diagnosed and, if you have suddenly found yourself in this position, to provide you with strategies to successfully survive and thrive in your role.

Watching a loved one go through pain and suffering causes excruciating, heart-wrenching emotional agony. The journey of a family member or friend of the diagnosed person can be just as emotionally traumatic as for the cancer patient.

As a parent, I watched both of my children, as newborns, fight to survive. I still remember the sleepless nights, vigilantly listening to my son's raspy breath for signs of deterioration, knowing he would likely get to the point when the arsenal of medication I had at home was not enough and we needed to go to the hospital, usually in the middle of the night. I would have traded places with him in an instant. I remember thinking, "Do whatever you want with me, but let my baby be healthy." The feeling of utter helplessness, the worry and anxiety over their prognosis…this is something you cannot truly understand unless you have been in a similar position.

1. EMOTIONAL STRESS

It is normal for a cancer patient's close family and friends to feel strong emotions when the cancer wrecking ball hits your world. There are many feelings and life changes that you need to cope with.

i. Helplessness

There is nothing more frustrating than the feeling of helplessness when you are sitting beside a loved one in great pain. If you have done everything you can to ensure their best care, then accept that there is nothing more you can do but be there for them.

ii. Worry and Anxiety

When you are supporting them in the fight of their life, your own worry and anxiety for them can seem insignificant and self-indulgent. It is not. You need to process and deal with your emotions in order to provide the stalwart support that your loved one needs.

iii. Loss

If your loved one is diagnosed with cancer, despite the most positive prognosis, it is natural for our minds to go to the worst-case scenario— the loss of our loved one. How will you live without them? What will happen to all the plans and dreams you had together? You may experience sadness and grief and may not even acknowledge these valid feelings because you are so busy trying to uplift the diagnosed person.

iv. Extra Load

Life goes on, even when someone has cancer. If your partner is suddenly hospitalised for treatment over weeks and months, children still need to be cared for, businesses need to be run, all the commitments that the cancer patient had before their diagnosis still have to be fulfilled.

What do you do when you work full-time and your wife is dealing with cancer treatment? How do you take on all her responsibilities and still fulfil your commitments to your job or business? Not only are you trying to manage two people's role, but you are doing it under the stress and worry about the impact on your children and the prognosis of your wife. And on top of that, you may also need to become a carer because when she is discharged from hospital, she may not be able to even walk up the stairs. How do you cope?

2. STRATEGY - "PUT ON YOUR OXYGEN MASK FIRST"

If you are a frequent flyer, you will have heard the safety instructions to put on your own oxygen mask before you help others. Why? Because if you run out of oxygen, you cannot help anyone else. If you are going to be able to help someone else, you need to get your oxygen mask on and be functioning at full capacity in order to be of service.

You need to first deal with your own unresolved emotions about the way cancer has upset your entire family's life. If you are the cancer patient's partner or their main carer, you may need help to process your personal emotional trauma.

Perhaps you are a strong and resilient person. You may be someone who can compartmentalise your feelings and tuck them away. I encourage you to instead deal with them, so you can be clearer mentally and emotionally in handling the situation.

Find a confidante, a person with whom you can share the load. Even the act of verbalising your thoughts can help activate that part of your brain which helps you to process your thoughts. Here are some suggestions that may help you:

i. Counselling

Seek a counsellor. You can contact your relevant cancer organisation or get a recommendation from your GP

ii. Journal/Blog

Write a journal of your thoughts to help you process the situation.

iii. Wellbeing

Keep yourself healthy by making good eating choices, getting enough sleep, exercising and staying grounded.

If you take steps to ensure your own wellbeing, it will be evident in the way you care for your loved one undergoing cancer treatment. Knowing that you are coping and that you are being supported is one of the best things you can do for them. It means that they can stop worrying about you and focus all their energy on healing themselves.

3. YOU ARE NOT ALONE

The cancer community is exceedingly kind. They say it takes a village to raise a child. I say that it takes a community to survive cancer.

i. Accept Help

Whether by word of mouth, the gossip grapevine or social media, everyone from your close family to casual acquaintances will know that cancer has impacted your family.

Messages of support and offers of assistance will probably come to you from everywhere. Sometimes we feel that it is our problem to deal with and we kindly smile and thank them for offering, and that is the end of it. Society used to be more community-based. Families lived in close proximity and extended family was always available to help. Since society has moved to the nuclear family model, often in different states or even different countries, this model has created an attitude where people feel like they need to deal with their problems on their own. But it does not have to be like that.

The story of Catur is a wonderful example of support from a global community. Catur and Sarah had run a successful business and were used to handling all their challenges on their own. When offers of support came in to Sarah during Catur's treatment, she eventually realised that she did not have the resources to go it alone. Sarah swallowed her pride and ego and accepted the love and support being offered. The generous help provided in services, time and monetary gifts spread the enormous load that had landed on her shoulders and allowed her to care for the love of her life while many of the practical things were taken care of.

One of the most important lessons that Sarah learned was that by gratefully receiving, she allowed her supporters to feel the beautiful joy of giving.

ii. Seek Help

Not everyone has a large network of friends, family and acquaintances. Perhaps you are new to an area and have not yet developed friendships. I encourage you to reach out and get the support you need. Contact your relevant cancer organisation to find out what support services they can offer to help you cope while you are caring for your loved one.

Many of these organisations have a vast range of services from emotional support staff through to practical assistance with transport. They understand that cancer is like a heavy stone dropped into a still lake. The impact causes a ripple effect, with the greatest intensity nearest the point of origin.

As the support person, you are closest to impact and these organisations understand that you need support too. Do not be embarrassed or ashamed to ask for counselling or assistance. You will be amazed at the help that will come flooding your way.

28

FOR THE PRIMARY SUPPORT PERSON:
HOW TO BE A GREAT CAREGIVER

THE STRESS OF SUDDENLY BEING THRUST INTO THE ROLE OF SUPPORT person may have you reaching for a cape and wishing for superpowers so you can be in two places at once, or at the very least, fly.

But you will not need super powers to be the best support person for your loved one. From talking to many cancer survivors and their support people, the key to great support comes down to a few simple things:

1. BE PRESENT

Just knowing you are there for me means everything. I do not expect you to take away my pain. I just need to know that when I need to talk to you and to lean on you, that you are there to hear me. Even when I am sick in a hospital bed, too weak to lift my head, knowing that you are beside me means more than I can say.

Sometimes I will ask you to come with me to appointments and treatments. Other times, I may need to be alone. Do not be offended if there are times when I need to be alone, because I need to process what is happening to me. And maybe, I do not want you to see when I feel weak and need to cry.

When I have side-effects like chemo brain, or exhaustion, or nerve pain, I may ask you for help or I may suffer in silence. Please do not suffocate me or tell me what I need. Please do not make me feel like a burden because of all the extra things you need to do. It will only make me feel worse.

Instead, please make it a safe place for me to be honest with you about how I feel and what I need. Open, non-judgemental communication will help me get through this crisis in the best way possible.

2. BE POSITIVE

The biggest worry that I have is the effect of my cancer diagnosis on you. Those of us who are parents of young children worry that they will be scared, and we who have older children worry that we might not be around to help them. We worry about our partners having to cope with continuing to go to work and cope with the added burden of taking care of the kids, the household and caring for us. We often spend more time worrying about everyone else besides ourselves.

One of the greatest things you can do is to handle all the stuff of life and be calmly positive. If I see that you are coping well and that you are confident and sure about my best outcome, that gives me a huge and uplifting boost. I can stop wasting my energy worrying if the dog has been fed, or that the kids have packed lunches. Your belief in my recovery is contagious and it keeps me moving in the right direction.

3. BE THE GATEKEEPER

This is something that can really help me to focus on recovery. Being a gatekeeper means discerning what needs my attention and what does not. If the matter is something you can take care of, then please do. If I am in hospital having chemo and the electricity bill needs to be paid, please do it. As a gatekeeper, you can keep friends and family informed so I do not have to be on social media and answering messages all day. There are some days when I would love to see people and other days when it is too much effort to talk. On those days, it would be so wonderful if you could explain why it might be better to see me on another day. If I have just had chemo and my white cell count is low, please check that visitors are healthy, so I do not get a virus that could be devastating to my health.

4. BE KNOWLEDGEABLE

Being fully briefed on my medical history and up-to-date with current treatment is vitally helpful to me. Keeping records and asking questions of my medical team when I am overwhelmed or cannot remember is so beneficial. Knowing that you have all the facts means I can discuss all my important medical decisions with you and that is of infinite value to me.

5. BE A RESEARCHER

Doctors, cancer survivors, support organisations, friends and family may make recommendations of therapies or other resources to help in my recovery. Some of these might be helpful and others may not. Support with investigating these suggestions is much appreciated.

You are the unsung hero of cancer survival. You are thanked, loved and appreciated for everything you do.

29

FOR THE PATIENT: SURVIVORSHIP

RESEARCH BREAKTHROUGHS AND ADVANCES IN MEDICAL TREATMENT have dramatically changed the outcomes for people diagnosed with cancer.

According to the U.S. National Cancer Institute, 62% of cancer survivors in the U.S. are currently 65 years of age or older, with estimates that by 2040, this figure will increase to 73%.

The Australian Institute of Health and Welfare reports similar rates of survivorship for Australians, with 68% cancer survival (based on data from 2009–2013) and estimates of 80% survivorship in 2017.

These statistics show that today, the majority of people survive cancer and go on to live for many years after their cancer treatment has ended. For some, transitioning from patient to survivor can be easy; for others, it can be just as challenging as the treatment. The stories you have read show that cancer affects everyone differently. Some people returned to their normal lives while others struggled to find their 'new normal.' Here are some of the things that helped me and the survivors in this book to thrive.

1. RE-ADJUST

We often use military words to describe our relationship to cancer. We use expressions that refer to cancer as 'a battle' or 'a fight for our life.' Our white blood cells are 'in a war' against the cancer cells and chemotherapy is like the atomic bomb that wipes out the enemies as well as the friendlies.

The analogy also works well to understand survivorship. There are plenty of books, movies and TV series that tell the story of soldiers, who spend months and sometimes years in battle, then struggle to adjust when they return to their previous life with home and family.

While soldiers are away in the armed forces, the chain of command means that the decision-making is taken out of their hands, and they must simply follow orders. This is similar to our time in cancer treatment. We are sent to tests by doctors, referred to specialists, and administered chemotherapy, We know we are under the care of experts, so we follow 'doctor's orders.'

While a soldier is fighting for his country, he may think often of his beautiful wife and children waiting at home for him, and long to be with them. Once he is actually home, it may be difficult to realign his instincts that have been finely tuned to be on guard for signs of the enemy. He may jump at the sound of a car backfiring or the loud noises of his children playing in the yard. We call it post-traumatic stress disorder (PTSD) and it is as relevant to cancer survivors as it is to soldiers.

Once your doctor pronounces that you are cancer-free and says you are in remission, you may have mixed feelings.

2. NOW WHAT?

After following your doctor's orders for so long, you may feel like a kite that has had its tether cut and is are now floating off into space. All that support that was holding your string taut has let go because your tribe thinks you are fine now and no longer need support. The truth is that you may feel more lost than ever, not wanting or able to go back to your previous work, or too battle weary to even try.

. . .

You may be asking yourself some of these questions:
"Why don't I feel better physically or emotionally?"
"Why don't I feel ecstatic that my treatment is over?"
"Why do I feel uncertain about my future?"
"Why can't I do what I used to?"
"Why do I feel so alone?"
"What if my cancer comes back?"

This is normal. You have been through a major, traumatic experience. Humans are not light switches—if we are in a dark place where our life is threatened, we cannot become instantly relaxed if you put us in the light amongst sunshine and rainbows.

Be gentle with yourself. Allow time to move at your own pace. Readjusting to life is a step that is part of your recovery. What can you do to make it easier?

i. Communicate

Tell your friends and family how you feel. Help them to understand what you are going through. You may look healthy and well, so they may not realise that you are still dealing with ongoing treatment symptoms that can often continue on after treatment, or that you are still dealing with emotional issues.

ii. Ask for Help

After treatment, you may experience long-term or irreversible changes to your body and the way it functions. You may have required surgery and need to adapt to the loss of body parts. You may have experienced other physical changes such as hair loss, weight gain, bladder or bowel changes. Hearing loss, mobility issues, early menopause, sexual and fertility changes are some of the other problems that can occur.

Talk to your doctor about ways to cope with these changes. There are specialists who can help you to adapt and to find new ways to live your life. Physiotherapists can help you with mobility, aids can improve hearing, fertility can be addressed with IVF.

Talk to your counsellor or psychologist and keep on with your sessions. Ask the people who supported you through your journey to stay close as you move through this phase of your recovery. Stay connected with your support group. This is probably the most important time to maintain your contact and involvement because these are people who have experienced exactly what you are going through and will be able to offer the wisdom of their experience.

iii. Keep up Your New Habits

If you have started some of the new habits discussed in previous chapters, keep them up. Continue your meditation and relaxation practices. Add to your journal every day, including a gratitude statement. Continue to read stories of cancer survivors, read positive books and material and watch uplifting shows and films. Laugh with friends. Increase your exercise a little each day. Resist the temptation to fall back into bad eating habits and strive for healthy meals and snacks.

iv. Hope

Nurture your mindset. Positive and hopeful thoughts are key to helping you to fully recover. Keep hope alive by fanning the flames to keep it blazing like a roaring fire. Hope is the light that shines like a beacon to guide us through the worst of experiences.

Sometimes our ability to keep the fires of hope burning brightly is compromised with fear and anxiety. One of the most common worries is that the cancer will return.

For many of us, this fear can become stronger when we are waiting for the results of our latest test. Anxiety can increase on particular dates such as the anniversary of diagnosis, or news of the death of someone with the same type of cancer as ours.

A practical way to set your mind at ease is to work out a follow-up care plan as soon as you are in remission. Arrange your next scan or check-up appointment. Ask your doctor for any symptoms you should look out for that might indicate a need for an earlier appointment. You can also compare notes with other people in your support group to find out the progress of their survivorship. The ladies in the Encore Group are a perfect example of how well this can work.

You do not have to deal with this alone. If your feelings of hopelessness are overwhelming you and you are depressed or frightened about the future, please talk to your GP and counsellor and ask for their help and advice. It is important to go to your doctor to check your symptoms, and they can help you get the assistance you need.

3. RE-EVALUATE

When we are struck by a life-changing, traumatic event, it is likely to cause us to re-evaluate the way we have been living our lives. Goals that we were working so hard to achieve may now seem less important.

Surviving cancer can feel like a second chance at life. Treat it like an opportunity rather than a frustration. Why wait until you are dying to come to the realisation that you have not lived a more fulfilling life? Are you living a life true to yourself? Are you communicating your true feelings? Do you have a supportive social circle of friends? What parts of your life really matter to you? Are you happy?

If you answered "no" to any of these questions, then have the courage to change. My life was irrevocably impacted by cancer. I re-evaluated my life and wondered why I was working just to earn money to live instead of doing the one thing I had always dreamed of doing since childhood—writing and speaking to inspire others.

You have within your hands the chance to design the way you want your world to be. Live without regret, change your life and the lives of others.

4. NEW PRIORITIES

After re-evaluating your life, you may set new priorities. Many of the people in this book realised that their family was their first priority and they changed their schedules, attitude and actions to truly reflect this. Others decided that life was too short to keep putting off their bucket list of adventures and they made the time to travel and to try new activities. Others realised that exercise and health required a higher priority in their life for them to feel happy and less stressed, and some realised that communicating their true feelings and speaking up for themselves was important in improving their relationships.

It is easy to get set on a path from a young age and to just "fall into" a career or job due to circumstances. If you love what you do, then surviving cancer will help you do it with a greater vision and perspective. If you find that you wish you were doing something else, then seek out ways to incorporate it into your life. The joy of doing what you love provides a level of satisfaction and happiness that will have you wishing you had explored it earlier!

5. GIVE BACK

A proven way to stop worrying about your own problems is to take the focus off you and to redirect it to someone or something else. Helping and learning about what others have been through certainly provides perspective on our own situation and can alter our outlook.

As a cancer survivor, you have so much to offer in terms of inspiring others with your story, assisting individuals, and contributing to causes that can make a huge difference to the world.

i. Mentor

Just as you may have benefited from the wisdom of a mentor or support group member during your cancer journey, so you can provide your perspective and encouragement to someone else going through a similar situation. From my experience and that of others who have been mentors, the joy and fulfilment in helping someone else provides immense satisfaction to both the giver and receiver.

ii. Volunteer, Fundraise, Donate

The cancer community is caring and inclusive. As a cancer patient, you may or may not have taken advantage of the services offered by the many organisations who provide emotional and practical support, survivorship services or research funding. Globally, there are too many foundations and institutes to list. If you have yet to connect to an organisation, explore your local area and contact the group toward which you feel affinity.

Fundraising to provide these services is always needed, and you can get involved at whatever level you choose. You may wish to donate financially, offer your time as a volunteer, or become involved in fundraising events. It is a great way to meet and associate with positive people, and to contribute to the universal goal of curing the disease once and for all.

THE SURVIVE AND THRIVE! SERIES

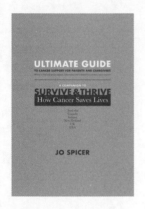

Ultimate Guide to Cancer Support for Patients and Caregivers is an essential resource for every cancer patient.

Part 1: Tips for patients and caregivers

Part 2: Directory of over 400 cancer support organisations and groups

Part 3: My Cancer Journey Workbook. AUD$19.95. www.jospicer.com

My Cancer Journey Workbook is a step-by-step workbook to guide you through your entire journey. Accurately record all of your doctors' appointments, medication, treatment protocols and more. Keeps vital details in one place for easy reference. For your FREE download and more information go to www.jospicer.com.

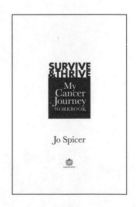

AFTERWORD

I hope that this book has given you a greater understanding of the ways in which cancer can impact a person's world. Everyone who has contributed their story has faced trauma, and in some cases, life-threatening disease, and survived.

No one in the book is a medical professional. We share our stories with the simple purpose of providing inspiration and hope for anyone who is experiencing life challenges.

When each of us faced our crisis, we determined that we would survive. Not every decision was the right one. Some caused setbacks. We experienced procedures that were excruciatingly painful and test results that turned our lives upside-down.

Each of us dealt with the situation in our own way. Our range of choices illustrate that there are no right or wrong ways to battle cancer; the key is to be informed of your options.

We hope our stories help you on your journey. We wish you effective treatment and wellness as you strive to survive and thrive!

ACKNOWLEDGEMENTS

This book was made possible through the generosity of all the people who shared their stories. My heartfelt thanks go out to each and every one of you. I feel so privileged to know you and am honoured by the trust you have given me.

My thanks also go my daughter, Brielle, who helped me to transcribe many of the interviews. We have supported each other through everything that life has presented. I am here for you no matter what. I love you and am privileged to be your mother.

My personal health journey, that ultimately led to the writing of this book, began during pregnancy with my son. Jadin, you had such a difficult and traumatic beginning and yet you have grown into an accomplished young man who I deeply admire and respect. I love you always.

The absolutely brilliant book cover is the design genius of my sister, Kerri Long. For our entire lives, we have been the yin and yang of creativity. You are the artist, I am the wordsmith. Your prowess in calligraphy and graphic design is astounding to me. I value your talents immensely and our sisterhood even more.

Perfection in spelling and grammar is something I continually strive to achieve. Maggie Ramsay has freely given of her time and expertise to ensure my passionate words are also grammatically correct. Maggie, your professional help and wholehearted support for this project has helped bring it to fruition.

Thanks also goes to Dr Eishitha Perera, who has kindly checked my medical terminology. Eisha, we are now family.

Liz Lobb, reconnecting after 30 years was wonderful. We picked up where we left off, as if those 30 years did not exist. Thank you for writing the foreword and for giving your time and support to this project.

Thank you all for helping me to bring this book to life. My wish is that it will inspire, uplift and provide hope when things seem the darkest. At those times, reading these stories of thriving survivors can help us all to keep hope alive.

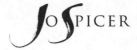

TERMINOLOGY INDEX

Various medical terms are used in this book. Here are some simple explanations to enhance your understanding.

Amniocentesis
A medical procedure used in prenatal diagnosis to check for abnormalities in the developing fetus (or foetus). A sample of amniotic fluid is drawn through a hollow needle inserted into the uterus.

Anti-Mullerian Hormone (AMH)
A hormone secreted by cells in developing egg sacs (follicles). The level of AMH in a woman's blood is generally a good indicator of her ovarian reserve.

Asperger's Syndrome
A developmental disorder affecting ability to effectively socialise and communicate.

Bilirubin
The yellow pigment created by the breakdown of red blood cells.

Bilateral Toe Fusion
Surgery to fuse both big toe joints.

Biopsy
A biopsy is a procedure to remove a piece of tissue or sample of cells

from the body for analysis in a laboratory. There are various types of biopsy procedures used in cancer diagnosis:

- **Bone Marrow Biopsy**: A sample of bone marrow is drawn from out of the back of your hipbone using a long needle.
- **Endoscopic Biopsy**: Used to collect samples from your internal organs, this type of biopsy uses a thin, flexible tube (endoscope) with a light on the end and special tools are passed through the tube to obtain the sample.
- **Needle Biopsy**: Procedure to obtain a sample of tissue or fluid from muscles, bones or other organs such as liver, thyroid and lungs.
- **Skin Biopsy:** Commonly used to diagnose melanoma. Cells are removed from the surface of your body.
- **Surgical Biopsy**: If the cells cannot be accessed by any other biopsy procedure, or if the results are inconclusive, a surgical biopsy may be required. An incisional biopsy is the removal of part of the abnormal area of cells, while an excisional biopsy removes the entire area of abnormal cells.

Blood Exchange Transfusion
A procedure to remove a person's entire blood supply and and replace it with fresh donor blood or plasma.
BMI
Body Mass Index. A measure of body fat based on your weight in relation to your height.
BRCA Gene
Mutations in BRCA 1 and BRCA 2 genes are associated with a higher risk of breast cancers.
Carcinoma
Cancer that begins in the skin or in tissue that lines or covers body organs. This can occur in the breast, colon, liver, lung, pancreas, prostate or stomach.
Catheter
A tube inserted into the bladder to drain urine from the body.

Cerebrospinal Fluid
Clear, colourless liquid that fills and surrounds the brain and the spinal cord and provides a mechanical barrier against shock.

Cervical Intraepithelial Neoplasia 3 (CIN3)
Severely abnormal growth of cells affecting the full thickness of the cervix. Also called high-grade or severe dysplasia.

Crohn's Disease
A chronic inflammatory disease of the digestive system including the mouth, intestines, colon and bowel.

CT Scan
Also known as a CAT scan or Computerised Axial Tomography. This is an X-ray test that produces cross-sectional images of the body using X-rays and computer technology. It allows the doctor to look inside the body in a similar way as you could look at a loaf of bread by slicing it. Think of it as a special type of X-ray that takes pictures of each slice of the body so that the doctor can look right at the area of interest. CT scans are frequently used to evaluate the brain, neck, spine, chest, abdomen, pelvis and sinuses.

Colonics
A colonic is the infusion of water into the rectum to cleanse and flush out the colon. It is also known as colonic hydrotherapy or colon irrigation and involves the continuous flow of water.

Colonoscopy
A procedure to visually examine the interior of the bowel. It. is performed on an empty bowel to check the bowel lining for changes.

Cryotherapy
The use of liquid nitrogen to freeze and kill cancer cells.

Cystectomy
The surgical removal of the bladder.

Digital Tomosynthesis
A three-dimensional mammogram.

Doctor
The term Doctor is interchangeable with Physician. As this book is written from an Australian perspective, I have utilised the more commonly-used word in this country being doctor.

Ductal

When used in conjunction with the word carcinoma, refers to cancer inside a milk duct. This is the most common form of breast cancer.

Dyspraxia
A childhood developmental disorder of the brain causing difficulty in activities requiring coordination and movement.

Endometriosis
A condition where endometrial tissue grows outside the uterus.

Enema
An injection of a liquid through the rectum to relieve constipation, for bowel cleansing or for diagnostic purposes (such as in a barium enema). Substances can be added to increase efficacy such as coffee, milk, saline or mineral oil.

Fibromyalgia
Widespread musculoskeletal (muscles and bones) chronic pain accompanied by fatigue, sleep, memory and mood issues. This condition amplifies painful sensations by affecting the way the brain processes pain signals.

Fistula
An abnormal connection or passageway that connects two organs that do not usually connect.

Gallium Scan
A diagnostic test where the radioactive metal gallium is injected into the body to identify infection, inflammation and tumours.

GP
Australia, NZ, Europe and UK, refer to the family doctor as a General Practitioner. In the USA and Canada, this would be equivalent to Family Physician (FP) or Family Medicine (FM).

Hemochromatosis
A condition where the body has too much iron.

HER2-Positive
This is a type of breast cancer that tests positive for a protein called human epidermal growth factor receptor 2 (HER2) which promotes the growth of cancer cells.

Hyperthermic Intraperitoneal Chemotherapy (HIPEC)
A treatment delivered in the form of a liquid to the abdominal cavity where it is heated to a temperature greater than normal body

temperature. The heat makes it more effective at killing the cancer cells and also improves blood flow within the abdominal cavity. This aids the delivery of chemotherapy to the cancer cells.

Hypothyroidism
A condition where the thyroid gland is underactive and does not produce enough thyroid hormones to meet the needs of the body.

Intensive Care Unit (ICU)
A unit of the hospital where seriously ill patients are cared for by doctors and nurses are specially trained in critical care.

Ileostomy
A pouch worn externally that is connected to your stomach to catch your digested food.

In Utero
In the womb.

IV Cannula
A thin tube inserted into a vein to administer medication, fluid, blood products or insert a surgical instrument.

In Vitro Fertilisation (IVF)
A medical procedure whereby an egg is fertilised by sperm, outside of the body, in a laboratory. The embryo is grown in a protected environment before being transferred into the woman's uterus to continue development.

Kidney Dialysis
When the kidneys can no longer function, dialysis replaces some of the functions by filtering the blood and removing waste, chemicals and fluid through an external dialysis machine.

Laser Therapy
A powerful beam of light used destroys cancerous cells.

Large Loop Excision of the Transformation Zone
A procedure to remove a small segment of the cervix.

Lobectomy
The surgical removal of a lobe of the lung.

Lumbar Puncture
The procedure of taking fluid from the spine in the lower back through a hollow needle, usually done for diagnostic testing.

Lupus
An autoimmune disease that can affect skin, joints, kidneys, heart

and lungs.

Lymphatic System
A network of vessels and organs throughout the whole body, which drains out toxins and cellular waste products and plays an important role in the immune responses.

Lymphoedema
This is the swelling of an arm or leg caused by a blockage in the lymphatic system. Can also be correctly spelled as lymphodema or lymphedema.

Lymphoma
Lymphoma is a condition when the lymphocytes (white blood cells that help to fight infection) become out of control. The lymphatic system runs throughout the body, including lymph nodes and organs and is part of the immune system. There are different types of lymphoma:

- **Burkitt's Lymphoma**: A rare but highly aggressive cancer that affects the mediastinum (chest), abdomen, central nervous system and vital organs. Common symptoms are swollen lymph nodes and abdominal swelling. It is a sub-category of B-cell Non-Hodgkin's Lymphoma.
- **Extra Nodal Marginal Zone Lymphoma**: Occurs outside of the lymph nodes and is a sub-category of B-cell Non-Hodgkin's Lymphoma.
- **Hodgkin's Lymphoma**: Distinguished by the presence of a cancer cell called a Reed-Sternberg cell. It often presents in the neck, under the arm or in the groin.
- **Primary Mediastinal B Cell Lymphoma**: A rare lymphoma affecting mainly young adults. It is aggressive and develops in the mediastinum (chest) and is a sub-category of Non-Hodgkin's Lymphoma.

Lymphoscintigram
A scan using a radioactive dye injected into the body to identify the closest draining lymph node to a breast tumour.

Mastectomy
Surgical removal of one whole breast.

Melanoma
A type of skin cancer where there is malignant transformation of melanocytes (the skin's pigment cells). When melanocyte cells aggregate together in the skin they form a mole, most of which are safe, but sometimes they can become a melanoma.

Metastatic
Cancer that spreads from the initial or primary site to other parts of the body by way of the blood or lymphatic vessels or membranous surfaces.

Muscular Dystrophy
A genetic disease that causes progressive weakness and loss of muscle mass.

Neobladder
A new bladder constructed to replace a removed non-functioning bladder. It is created from a piece of intestine that is reconstructed to form the new (neo) bladder.

Nephrectomy
The surgical removal of one or both kidneys.

Neuroendocrine Tumour
Rare tumours that develop in the cells of the nerves (neuro) in the endocrine system (the network of glands and organs in the body that produces hormones). Neuroendocrine tumours (NETS) arise from neuroendocrine cells, which are cells that release hormones into the blood in response to a neuron signal. They commonly occur in the intestine, but are also found in the pancreas, lung and other organs.

Neutropenic
A condition where one has an abnormally low count of white blood cells.

Oophorectomy
The surgical removal of ovaries.

Percutaneous Endoscopic Gastrostomy (P.E.G.)
A surgical procedure to insert a feeding tube through the skin and into the stomach. It is used for people who have trouble swallowing or eating sufficient food and drink.

Peritoneum
The thin, delicate sheet that lines the inside wall of the abdomen and is made of epithelial cells.

PET Scan
Positron Emission Tomography. A nuclear medicine imaging test where a radioactive liquid, fluorodeoxyglucose (a simple sugar substance), is injected into the bloodstream. The liquid accumulates in the parts of the body that gives off gamma rays and are detected by the PET scanner and a computer converts the signals in to images. This is commonly used for cancer imaging because cancer cells are rapidly dividing cells that needs sugar for growth.

Phototherapy
Special lighting that emits rays in the blue-green spectrum.

PICC
A peripherally inserted central catheter.

Portacath
Implanted venous (veins) access device for patients who require the frequent or continuous administration of chemotherapy. It consists of a reservoir (the port) and a tube (the catheter). The port is implanted under the skin, usually in the upper chest, and attached to the catheter that is threaded into a large vein.

Postpartum Thyroiditis
An inflammation of the thyroid gland that occurs after pregnancy.

Pseudomyxoma Peritonei Cancer
A rare cancer that makes a jelly-like liquid called mucin. It spreads into the space inside the peritoneum (layers of tissue that lines the abdomen). As the mucin builds, it puts pressure on the bowel and other organs.

Post-Traumatic Stress Disorder (PTSD)
A particular set of reactions that can develop in people who have been through a traumatic event that threatened their life or safety, or that of a close friend or relative. As a result, the person may experience intrusive symptoms of nightmares or anxiety when faced with traumatic reminders. Affected persons may also display avoidance behaviours and experience distress, isolation and functional impairment.

Quintuple Bypass Surgery
When all five of the major vessels to the heart are diseased, this surgery is performed.

Radical Mastectomy
A procedure where the entire breast is removed.
Radical Neck Dissection
Removal of lymph nodes from the neck.
Radiation Enteritis
Inflammation of the intestine due to radiation.
Retinoblastoma
An eye cancer that starts in the retina, the light-sensing area at the back of the eye. It usually occurs in young children under three years of age and can affect one or both eyes.
Shingles
A painful and acute rash caused by the same virus as chickenpox.
Specialist
This refers to a doctor who has trained further and received accreditation in a specific field such as Oncology, Obstetrics, Paediatrics etc.
Stem Cells
Cells in the body that have the potential to divide indefinitely and differentiate into specific cell types.
Stoma
An artificial opening on the wall of the abdomen with a bag attached to collect waste.
Superficial Parotidectomy
Removal of his major and largest salivary gland.
Thoracotomy
A major surgical procedure where an incision is made into the pleural space of the chest.
Total Pelvic Exenteration
Surgery that removes the bladder, urethra, large intestine, rectum, anus, ovaries, fallopian tubes, uterus and vagina.
Transverse Rectus Abdominus Musculocutaneous Flap (TRAM Flap)
A procedure where a flap of the abdominal skin, fat, and muscle are used to reconstruct the breasts.
Tubal ligation
A surgical procedure for female sterilization which involves clipping, cutting, tying or sealing shut the fallopian tubes.

Ureters

The tubes that carry urine from the kidneys to the urinary bladder. There are two ureters, one attached to each kidney. The upper half is located in the abdomen and the lower half is located in the pelvic area.

Urethra

The tube that connects the urinary bladder for the removal of urine from the body.

Urinary Tract Infection (UTI)

An infection in any part of the urinary system—kidneys, ureters, bladder or urethra.

Vascular Catheter

Collection of blood via a tube inserted into the femoral vein in the groin. This is performed as a day surgery procedure.

Vena Cava

The large vein from the heart to the lower part of the body.

Vesicoureteral Reflux

The backwards flow of urine from the bladder to the kidneys.

Vulval Intraepithelial Neoplasia (VIN)

Abnormal changes in the epithelial or surface layer of cells of the vulva.

Wide Local Excision

Surgery to cut out the cancer and some healthy tissue around it.

Wilms' Tumour

Also known as Nephroblastoma, this is a childhood kidney cancer that can affect both kidneys. It is believed to grow as the fetus (foetus) develops in the womb and hereditary.

ABOUT THE AUTHOR

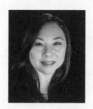

Jo's passion for writing began as a young child growing up in Sydney, Australia. An avid reader with an overactive imagination, Jo wrote her first fiction novel at the age of 10.

Intent on developing a career with words, Jo completed her degree in Journalism and Communications at the University of Technology and embarked on a 30-year career in writing, marketing, sales, training and public speaking.

Today Jo is the author of both non-fiction and fiction books in various genres including inspiration, wellness and self-development. She also writes romance, young adult urban fantasy and children's books.

Apart from her writing, Jo relishes good food, laughter, travel and time with family and friends. She loves reading fascinating stories in books, movies and TV series.

For FREE giveaways and more go to www.jospicer.com